MCQs in Obstetrics and Gynaecology

MCQs in Obstetrics and Gynaecology

John Studd
MD MRCOG
Consultant Obstetrician and Gynaecologist,
King's College Hospital and Dulwich Hospital, London

D M F Gibb
BSc MRCP MRCOG
Lecturer in Obstetrics and Gynaecology, University of Singapore, Kandang
Kerbau Hospital for Women, Singapore

Churchill Livingstone
EDINBURGH LONDON MELBOURNE AND NEW YORK 1983

Medical Division of Longman Group UK Limited

Distributed in the United States of America by Churchill
Livingstone Inc., 1560 Broadway, New York, N.Y. 10036,
and by associated companies, branches and
representatives throughout the world.

First published 1983
  Reprinted 1984
  Reprinted 1988

ISBN 0 443 02283 6

British Library Cataloguing in Publication Data
Studd, John W. W.
  MCQs in obstetrics and gynaecology.
  1. Gynecology — Examinations, questions, etc.
  2. Obstetrics — Examinations, questions, etc.
  I. Title   II. Gibb D. M.
  618'.076   RG111

Library of Congress Cataloguing in Publication Data
Studd, John.
  MCQs in obstetrics and gynaecology.
  Bibliography: p.
  1. Obstetrics — Examinations, questions, etc.
  2. Gynecology — Examinations, questions, etc. I. Gibb,
  D. M. F. II. Title. [DNLM: 1. Gynecology — Examination
  questions. 2. Obstetrics — Examination questions.
  WQ 18 S933m]
  RG111.S88   1983   618'.076   82–14694

Produced by Longman Singapore Publishers Pte Ltd
Printed in Singapore

Preface

Multiple choice questions have become firmly established in examinations. They have been used for many years in North America and are now increasingly used in Britain. The London Universities Board have introduced them into the obstetrics and gynaecology undergraduate examinations and the Royal College of Obstetricians and Gynaecologists uses them in Part I and Part II of the Membership examination (MRCOG).

The stimulus to their wider use has been the desire for greater objectivity and fairness and the availability of sophisticated technology to facilitate consistent and rapid marking. The main part of the MRCOG written examination remains as essay questions, as the ability to discuss and develop arguments relevant to clinical situations must be assessed and this can only be expressed in essay-type answers. The much broader base of factual knowledge is better assessed by multiple choice questions. The clinical and viva voce parts of the examination retain their important place in overall assessment in an essentially clinical subject.

Candidates reading for examinations become concerned about whether time spent reading and rereading textbooks has been of real value in improving their knowledge. Rereading may be useful, but a method of determining what requires to be reread will lead to improved efficiency in revision. Answering multiple choice questions provides such a method and at the same time provides the student with a self-assessment of his knowledge and recognition of areas for further study. Familiarisation with the method is also important and this book may be used for trial runs and practice with the technique.

Some of the points of technique are illustrated in our questions and the pitfalls elaborated in the comment which we considered important to add to each answer in order to make the book a teaching aid. We have included references where we think they are important and the list of references constitutes a recommended further reading list. Some questions have been left with an open reference where the information is taken from various sources or where practical points are discussed, sometimes not having a clearly right or wrong answer. We thought it important to include such questions to stimulate discussion and deeper understanding of practical points. There may be a lack of general agreement about some answers. We expect this.

In an examination itself such questions might be considered unfair, but experience shows that only a small number of questions in the examination fall into this category. Whilst we have tried to set the questions at a level appropriate for postgraduate students preparing for the MRCOG examination, some questions are clearly much too difficult and some are much too easy.

London 1983

J W W S
D M F G

Contents

The multiple choice question

FORMAT OF QUESTIONS

A variety of formats have been tried but only one has become widely used in obstetrics and gynaecology in Britain. This format is the 'Multiple true/false' or 'determinant response' format. A common STEM is used followed by five independent ITEMS as shown in example 1. Each item should read in correct prose with the stem and the candidate is asked to determine whether the resulting STATEMENTS are true or false. Alternatively the stem may be used to introduce several statements which may be true or false.

Example 1
Amniotic fluid embolism
  A is usually fatal
  B characteristically presents before delivery
  C occurs more commonly in multiparous patients
  D is diagnosed by specific staining techniques
  E has been treated with heparin
The answers are usually clear-cut, but the ability of the candidate to answer will depend on how much he has read about the condition. (a) and (c) are true, being well documented in most texts, whilst (e) is true but that correct response will depend upon deeper reading. (d) is true and is used to direct the students attention to the difficulties of clinical diagnosis which may only be confirmed on post mortem examination. (b) is false and illustrates both the use of the word characteristic and the use of a direct opposite.

Terminology
Terminological conventions are important and words like 'characteristic', 'associated', 'typical' and 'recognized' must be interpreted literally. Each word should be carefully considered but problems should not be sought by excessive analysis which the examiner clearly did not consider. Esoteric knowledge is not relevant and the answer will depend on well-established wisdom found in recent texts. This should not be taken to mean that clearly established modern advances are excluded. A statement that something occurs in a certain disease does mean that it occurs all the time or that it occurs rarely, but that it occurs often enough to be associated with it.

Numbers must be scrutinized and the denominator is of as much importance as the numerator given in a rate. Words that look or sound similar may be used to mislead the candidate who has not read the question carefully. Simple tricks may be built into the question but more elaborate deceptions are unlikely.

It is evident that not all statements in medicine, especially in obstetrics and gynaecology are clearly true or false and there must be a grey area. This type of question will not be common in the exam, but we have used them as teaching points.

Examination technique
Whilst technique alone does not enable one to pass an exam, it may make a great difference, especially in a borderline case. A logical and clearly-defined approach is desirable.

An example of the mark-sense answer card for optico-electronic processing of the 'determinate response' type of MCQ is shown in Figure 1. Clear instructions about the use of a pencil to mark the card, how to fill in each box and how to document the candidates name and number must be meticulously respected. The true/false/don't know response is read by a computer and there is no place for discussion. The correct answer gains one mark, the wrong answer loses one mark and a 'don't know' response neither gains nor loses. Failure to mark the card in the correct way may lead to a 'don't know' response being recorded.

As in any examination reading the question carefully is of paramount importance. Scrutiny of the words used and underlining important points on the question sheet is useful. Any amount of writing or rough work is permissible on the question sheet and the answer should be initially written there. At the end of each question the candidate should transfer his considered response to the computer card. Care should be exercised in marking the computer card in pencil in the right direction at the end of each question. Leaving all responses to be transferred at the end of the examination is foolish as time may run out although questions are answered, the computer receives nothing.

The candidate must reflect on whether his knowledge allows him to answer a question. A truthful 'don't know' is preferable to a guess. It becomes clear that his response will be that a statement is clearly 'true', clearly 'false', possibly 'don't know' or definitely 'don't know'. It is advisable to mark the last category as 'don't know' but to assess objectively what the chance is of answering the possibly 'don't know' correctly. The desirability of answering such questions will also depend on how many other questions have been answered. There is a place for leaving some responses blank until the other questions have been answered. This is only appropriate for small number of questions or confusion may arise. It is possible to lower a mark that would have produced a pass by guessing and self-deception about the ability to answer is likely to lead to failure. Post graduates will be expected to score in range of 55–70%, but the pass mark will vary with each examination.

It is more difficult to set multiple choice questions than to answer them, and we must express our thanks to Mr David Oram, Mr Nick Siddell and Mr Malcolm Pearce for careful proof-reading and advice, which has removed ambiguities from the questions.

We have attempted to give a reference with each question, but as all 5 parts of a question may not be found within one reference, we have allowed ourselves the occasional license, when designating authorship of a statement. The references can be found at the rear of the book, and are a very personal, but incomplete, collection of recommended texts.

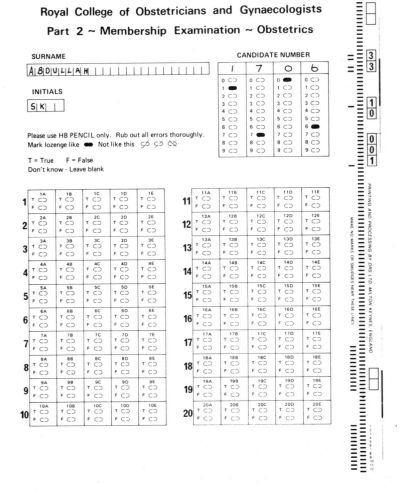

1. Obstetrics

1.1 The maternal mortality rate in England and Wales
  A is about 11 per 100 000 total maternities
  B includes women dying up to one year after childbirth
  C does not include women dying from the complications of ectopic pregnancy
  D is analysed in biennial reports of confidential enquiries
  E does not include deaths associated with abortion

1.2 The birth rate in England and Wales
  A is about 13 per 1000 female population
  B reached a peak in the mid 1960's
  C is rising
  D allows approximately zero population growth
  E was about four times the rate of termination of pregnancy in 1979

1.3 The perinatal mortality rate (PNMR) in England and Wales
  A is 25 per 1000 total births
  B is falling
  C is higher in lower socio-economic groups
  D reveals that prematurity is the most common cause of death
  E would be reduced much more by improved social conditions rather than electronic fetal heart rate monitoring

(*Answers overleaf*)

1.1 A **True**   Factual information derived from the Report on
     B **True**   Confidential Enquiries into Maternal Deaths is very
     C **False**   important. This is a detailed audit and analysis of the
     D **False**   most serious outcome of obstetric problems and
     E **True**   their management. It considers avoidable and
                    unavoidable factors and therefore makes
                    recommendation as to areas in which care could be
                    improved. It is published every three years and is
                    indispensable reading for postgraduate students.
                    Although deaths from abortion are analysed in the
                    Confidential enquiry they are not included in the
                    mortality rate because the denominator refers to total
                    births (which are registered) not to total pregnancies
                    (which are not registered).

Ref 1

1.2 A **False**   The birth rate is about 13 per 1000 *total home*
     B **True**   population. Although the number cited is correct the
     C **True**   denominator is incorrect and the statement is false.
     D **True**   This is a common trap for the unwary. Some
     E **True**   knowledge of the epidemiological background to
                    obstetrics is essential. At the time of writing (1981)
                    the birth rate is rising again. In most Western
                    countries the birth rate is approximately equal to the
                    death rate and this permits zero population growth
                    after correction for migration. In 1979 there were
                    about four times as many births as terminations of
                    pregnancy.

Refs 1 and 2

1.3 A **False**   At the time of writing the PNMR in England and
     B **True**   Wales is about 15 per 1000 total births and is falling.
     C **True**   Many of these babies are born prematurely and this
     D **True**   occurs more often in the lower socio-economic
     E **True**   groups. Prematurity, congenital abnormality and
                    birth asphyxia are the three main causes of perinatal
                    death. Electronic fetal heart rate monitoring has been
                    shown to have little effect on overall mortality,
                    although it may reduce death due to intrapartum
                    hypoxia in high risk labours.

G V P Chamberlain in Ref 3

1.4   International comparisons of perinatal mortality rates reveal that:
    A England and Wales has a higher perinatal mortality rate or PNMR than Scandinavia
    B England and Wales has a higher PNMR than Scotland
    C more cases of spina bifida occur in England and Wales than in France
    D England and Wales has a lower PNMR than USA
    E Holland has the best PNM figures in Europe

1.5   The confidential enquiry into maternal deaths, England & Wales 1973-75 (1979) reported that:
    A women of non-Caucasian origin were at a smaller risk of death from hypertension than Caucasian women
    B more women die of post-partum haemorrhage than ante-partum haemorrhage
    C pulmonary embolism was the most common cause of maternal death
    D the majority of uterine ruptures leading to maternal death were due to rupture or dehiscence of a previous scar
    E there were more deaths from coronary heart disease than from rheumatic heart disease

1.6   The confidential enquiry into maternal death, England and Wales 1973–75 (1979) reported that:
    A the fatality rate for Caesarean section in NHS patients is 1.9/1000 maternities
    B in deaths related to anaesthesia avoidable factors were present in 90%
    C antacids protect from Mendelson's syndrome
    D failed intubation at induction of anaesthesia was the most common primary anaesthetic factor
    E there were no deaths due to epidural analgesia during the three year study

1.7   Fertilization
    A occurs in the uterine cavity
    B if effected by two spermatozoa causes a trisomic conceptus
    C is associated with a surge of maternal luteinizing hormone
    D is associated with production of the first polar body
    E depends on hyaluronidase release by the sperm

(*Answers overleaf*)

1.4 A **True**   Sweden has the best perinatal results in Europe,
     B **False** followed by Denmark (1972). Holland has excellent
     C **True**   results (4th), and notable because of the large
     D **True**   number of home confinements. Scotland traditionally
     E **False** has had a worse perinatal rocord than England and
                  Wales, but the results have improved dramatically in
                  the last two years. Spina bifida is more common in
                  the British Isles (8–12/10 000) than anywhere in
                  Europe (1–2/10 000).

G Chamberlain in Ref 3

1.5 A **False** Hypertension is now the most common cause of
     B **True**   death, being a much greater risk in black women than
     C **False** white. There were far more deaths from post-partum
     D **False** haemorrhage than ante-partum haemorrhage and
     E **True**   uterine ruptures were more common than
                  dehiscence of the scar possibly because of the
                  increased use of oxytocics for induction and
                  augmentation of labour. Rheumatic heart disease is
                  now quite rare and the increased mortality from
                  coronary heart disease probably reflects differing
                  life-style and smoking habits in women.

Ref 1

1.6 A **False** The fatality rate for Caesarean section was 0.8/1000
     B **True**   being approximately 8–10 times that of a vaginal
     C **False** delivery. Unfortunately antacid therapy as presently
     D **False** practised does not protect from aspiration
     E **False** pneumonia as most patients in the report who had
                  died of this condition had received preinduction
                  antacids. Inhalation of stomach contents was the
                  most important primary anaesthetic factor (13
                  deaths) and failed intubation the second most
                  important (7 deaths). There were two deaths directly
                  attributable to epidural anaesthesia during the three
                  year study. The inexperience of the anaesthetist was
                  noted as being important.

Ref 1

1.7 A **False** Fertilization occurs in the outer part of the fallopian
     B **False** tube the conceptus then taking several days to travel
     C **False** to the uterine cavity. An ovum fertilized by more than
     D **False** one sperm results in polyploidy. There is no
     E **True**   associated maternal hormone change and
                  fertilization occurs at the time of formation of the
                  second polar body. Hyaluronidase released by the
                  sperm facilitates its penetration of the zona
                  pellucida.

E D Morris in Ref 4

1.8 In human placentation the following structures lie between maternal and fetal blood:
A chorion laeve
B decidua
C trophoblast
D capillary endothelium
E mesenchyme

1.9 The following statements about the placenta are correct:
A there is a close correlation between chorionic villous area and birth weight
B there is a close correlation between calcification and functional efficiency
C it produces acid phosphatase
D its barrier function is important
E the cytotrophoblastic cells have microvilli

1.10 Human chorionic gonadotrophin (HCG)
A is a glycoprotein
B is secreted by the trophoblast before implantation
C has a β subunit similar to follicle stimulating hormone (FSH)
D reaches a peak level at 20 weeks' gestation
E is involved in the induction of fetal testosterone secretion

1.11 The following statements concerning oestrogen metabolism in pregnancy are correct:
A the placenta synthesizes oestriol from pregnenolone
B qualitatively plasma oestriol levels are similar to urinary oestriol levels
C the fetal liver hydroxylates dehydro-epiandrosterone sulphate (DHAS)
D oestriol secretion increases throughout normal pregnancy
E fetal adrenal function is reflected in oestriol production.

1.12 The following maternal hormone changes are observed during normal pregnancy:
A increased luteinizing hormone (LH)
B increased aldosterone secretion
C increased secretion of oxytocin near term
D increase in plasma cortisol near term
E increase in plasma growth hormone

(*Answers overleaf*)

1.8 A **False**   In the haemochorial human placenta maternal blood
     B **False**   in the intervillous space bathes the villi which are
     C **True**   composed of syncytiotrophoblast, cytotrophoblast, a
     D **True**   mesenchymal core and contain fetal capillaries.
     E **True**

E D Morris in Ref 4

1.9 A **True**   There is a poor correlation between macroscopic
     B **False**   changes in the placenta and function. However,
     C **False**   chorionic villous area is proportional to placental and
     D **False**   birth weights. The placenta produces heat stable
     E **False**   alkaline phosphatase. The syncytio-trophoblast
                      possessing microvilli is involved in the transfer of
                      molecules and the postulated passive barrier
                      function is now not thought to be a significant
                      feature.

E D Morris in Ref 4

1.10 A **True**   HCG is a glycoprotein composed of α and β sub units.
     B **True**   The α sub units are also possessed by
     C **False**   thyroid-stimulating hormone, luteinizing hormone
     D **False**   (LH) and follicle stimulating hormone (FSH). The β
     E **True**   sub unit only shares characteristics with the β sub
                      unit of LH. Secretion reaches a peak at 14 weeks'
                      gestation and has fallen substantially by 20 weeks.
                      There is now evidence of its involvement in the
                      induction of fetal testosterone secretion.

E D Morris in Ref 4

1.11 A **False**   The complexity of oestrogen metabolism makes
     B **True**   estimation of oestriol production a poor reflection of
     C **True**   placental function. DHAS produced by the fetal
     D **True**   adrenal is hydroxylated in fetal liver and then
     E **True**   metabolized to oestriol in placental tissue. The
                      function of several organs and blood circulation is
                      involved. Maternal adrenal secretion of DHAS is also
                      thought to be important.

E D Morris in Ref 4

1.12 A **False**   FSH and LH are consistently depressed during
     B **True**   pregnancy while oestrogens, progesterone and
     C **False**   prolactin are increased. Oxytocin has not been
     D **True**   demonstrated to have a primary role in the onset of
     E **False**   spontaneous labour and probably acts secondarily to
                      prostaglandins. Cortisol is increased and fetal cortisol
                      may play a part in the onset of labour. Maternal
                      growth hormone secretion does not increase.

R P Shearman in Ref 4

1.13 The following biochemical changes relative to the non pregnant values are considered normal in a pregnant patient:
  A   elevated blood urea
  B   elevated alkaline phosphatase
  C   elevated fasting blood sugar
  D   decreased serum albumin
  E   elevated serum lipids

1.14 Asymptomatic bacteriuria
  A   occurs in 10% of pregnant women
  B   converts to overt infection in about 30% of untreated patients
  C   occurs in patients with renal tract abnormalities
  D   is associated with prematurity
  E   causes an increased white cell count

1.15 Smoking in pregnancy is associated with
  A   infants with low developmental quotient
  B   unemployment
  C   antenatal clinic non attendance
  D   decreased incidence of breast feeding
  E   increased incidence of pre eclampsia

1.16 When pregnancy is complicated by glycosuria
  A   a fasting blood sugar of greater than 8 mmol/l is diagnostic of diabetes mellitus.
  B   a fasting blood sugar of less than 6 mmol/l excludes diabetes mellitus.
  C   it is associated with decreased tubular re-absorption of glucose.
  D   a glucose tolerance test should be performed after one positive test for glycosuria.
  E   the patient has impaired glucose tolerance.

(*Answers overleaf*)

1.13 A **False**   Blood urea is usually decreased in the pregnant state
     B **True**   because of the raised glomerular filtration rate and
     C **False**   even a value in the upper limit of normal for the non
     D **True**   pregnant state would be considered abnormal.
     E **True**   Alkaline phosphatase is usually elevated in normal
pregnancy due to placental production and has been
used in the past as a test of placental function.
Fasting blood sugar is low, although response to a
glucose load may be impaired. Serum lipids are
commonly elevated and serum albumin decreased.

D A Davey in Ref 4

1.14 A **False**   Asymptomatic bacteriuria in pregnancy occurs in
     B **True**   approximately 5% of patients but is worth detecting
     C **True**   because about 30% of these may be expected to
     D **True**   convert to overt infection. There is also an
     E **False**   association with pregnancy complications such as
pre term labour. These patients may have structural
abnormalities of the urinary tract and if bacteriuria is
persistent an intravenous urogram should be
performed after delivery. Bacteria in the urine rarely
cause an increased white cell count unless the renal
substance is infected.

C J Dewhurst in Ref 4

1.15 A **True**   Smoking in pregnancy causes low birth weight
     B **True**   babies who subsequently have a lower IQ and DQ.
     C **True**   This social characteristic is a valuable marker of a
     D **True**   high risk pregnancy in that the patients are more
     E **False**   commonly unmarried, unemployed, unsure of dates,
do not breast feed and have greater problems with
care of the infant. There is some evidence that
pre-eclampsia is less common in smokers.

J Murphy in Ref 3 Vol 3

1.16 A **True**   Glycosuria on one occasion in the absence of a
     B **True**   suggestive history is not an indication for a glucose
     C **False**   tolerance test. Lowered renal threshold is a common
     D **False**   cause of glycosuria in pregnancy. Tubular
     E **False**   reabsorption of glucose remains unaltered, but the
amount of glucose in the glomerular filtrate
increases, and overflow therefore occurs.

J M Brudenell in Ref 3 Vol 2

1.17 The following statements about proteinuria in pregnancy are true:

A it is usually selective
B daily urinary protein loss increases progressively during pregnancy
C Esbach method is an adequate semi quantitative investigation
D if more than 2 g/day is most likely due to a urinary tract infection
E it contains Immunoglobulin G (IgG)

1.18 A 20 year old pregnant woman is found to have a haemoglobin of 9 g/dl, an MCV of 70 femtolitres, a mean cell haemoglobin concentration (MCHC) of 28 g/dl, a serum iron of 9 nanomoles/l and a total iron binding capacity (TIBC) of 106. You would expect this patient to have

A a microcytic blood film
B target cells on the blood film
C a high blood urea
D a reticulocyte count of approximately 10%
E a good response to folic acid therapy

1.19 Toxoplasmosis in a pregnant woman

A is caused by a bacterium
B is commonly asymptomatic
C causes choroidoretinitis in the fetus
D causes abortion
E causes cerebral calcification in the neonate

1.20 The following statements about carbohydrate metabolism are correct:

A Maturity-onset diabetics show no insulin response to a glucose load
B Tubular reabsorption of glucose is less efficient in pregnancy
C Normal women show progressive impairment of glucose intolerance in pregnancy
D There is increased glucose concentration in the glomerular filtrate in pregnancy
E Renal threshold rises with age

1.21 The following pregnancy complications are associated with well controlled diabetes mellitus:

A Spontaneous abortion
B Premature labour
C Hyperemesis
D Urinary tract infection
E Pre eclampsia

(Answers overleaf)

1.17 A **False**   The physiological daily protein loss is increased in
     B **True**   normal pregnancy from 0–5 mgs/100 ml to
     C **False**   5–10 mgs/100 ml in the last trimester, but these levels
     D **False**   are usually undetectable by standard clinical
     E **True**   methods. The proteinuria is nearly always poorly
                    selective, always contains Immunoglobulin G and if
                    due to urinary tract infection is rarely present in
                    excess of 2 g/day.

J W W Studd in Ref 5

1.18 A **True**   This patient with iron deficiency anaemia will have a
     B **False**   microcytic blood film and a reticulocyte count less
     C **False**   than 2%, with no target cells. Target cells are found in
     D **False**   haemolytic anaemias or liver disease. A high blood
     E **False**   urea would produce a normocytic normochromic
                    anaemia.

1.19 A **False**   Toxoplasmosis is caused by the protozoon
     B **True**   toxoplasma gondii. Infection is often asymptomatic
     C **True**   but fetal effects include abortion, choroidoretinitis,
     D **True**   cerebral calcification, jaundice and
     E **True**   hepatosplenomegaly.

E D Morris in Ref 4

1.20 A **False**   Carbohydrate metabolism is altered in pregnancy
     B **False**   with a lowered renal threshold leading to glycosuria
     C **True**   and impaired glucose tolerance. This is because of an
     D **False**   increased glomerular filtration rate with no extra
     E **True**   capacity of the tubules to absorb the excess glucose.
                    Maturity onset diabetics diabetics secrete insulin in
                    response to a glucose load although delayed and
                    exaggerated. Juvenile onset diabetics show no such
                    response. Renal threshold to sugar rises with age.

J M Brudenell in Ref 3 Vol 2

1.21 A **False**   Good control of maternal blood sugar is the key to
     B **True**   the management of diabetic pregnancy. Such cases
     C **False**   do not abort or suffer from hyperemesis gravidarum
     D **True**   more frequently than do controls, but they may have
     E **True**   pre eclampsia, urinary tract infection or hydramnios.
                    Premature labour is commoner in diabetic
                    pregnancy.

J M Brudenell in Ref 3 Vol 2

1.22 Babies born to diabetic mothers
  A   have an increased incidence of fetal abnormalities
  B   have an increased incidence of the caudal regression
       syndrome
  C   have an increased incidence of renal vein thrombosis
  D   if stillborn, may have hypoplasia of the islet cells of the
       pancreas
  E   are more commonly male than female

1.23 Good control of diabetes in pregnancy
  A   maintains blood sugar levels between 8 and 12 mmol/l
  B   is achieved by twice daily injections of insulin
  C   reduces the incidence of polyhydramnios
  D   reduces the incidence of congenital abnormalities
  E   is aimed a reducing fetal hyperinsulinism

**1.24 The following contribute to good control of diabetes in
pregnancy:**
  A   300 g carbohydrate per day diet
  B   good control of protein intake
  C   oral hypoglycaemic drugs in mild cases
  D   twice-daily mixtures of short and medium acting insulins
  E   elimination of infection

**1.25 The following statements about diabetes mellitus and
pregnancy are true:**
  A   The perinatal mortality is about 50/1000 with good care
  B   Intrauterine death is usually the result of placental
       insufficiency
  C   Control of diabetes should be maintained with a blood
       glycosylated haemoglobin of less than 12%
  D   Control of blood sugar reduces the incidence of fetal
       macrosomia
  E   The use of dexamethasone if the L/S ratio is low necessitates
       the administration of insulin.

(Answers overleaf)

1.22 A **True**   The baby of a diabetic mother shows characteristic
     B **True**   changes often related to the quality of maternal
     C **True**   blood glucose control. Poorly controlled diabetics
     D **False**   have big babies, big placentas and excess liquor.
     E **False**   Fetal abnormalities are four times as common even
                     with good control and the fetal abnormality of
                     agenesis of the sacrum and hypoplasia of the lower
                     limbs, (caudal regression syndrome) occurs rarely
                     although more often than in non diabetics. Post
                     mortem studies of stillborn babies show hyperplasia
                     of the islet cells of the pancreas.

J M Brudenell in Ref 3 Vol 2

1.23 A **False**   Many of the complications of diabetic pregnancy are
     B **True**   known to be related to poor control of blood sugar
     C **True**   levels which should be maintained below
     D **True**   10 mmol/l. 12 mmol/l is too high and a level may
     E **True**   often be below 8 mmol/l. This control necessitates
                     twice daily insulin injections with monitoring of
                     blood glucose rather than urinary glucose, which is
                     not adequate because of the altered renal threshold
                     in pregnancy. Fetal death in utero is probably due to
                     maternal hyperglycaemia producing fetal
                     hyperinsulinism and consequent hypoglycaemia. The
                     incidence of congenital abnormalities is reduced,
                     although not eliminated.

J M Brudenell in Ref 3 Vol 2

1.24 A **False**   Diabetic diet contains between 150 and 250 g of
     B **False**   carbohydrate per day and no restriction is placed on
     C **False**   fat or protein intake. Oral hypoglycaemic drugs do
     D **True**   not given good control and twice daily injections of
     E **True**   insulin are preferable. Infections precipitate
                     hyperglycaemia and should be eliminated.

J M Brudenell in Ref 3 Vol 2

1.25 A **True**   Even with good diabetic control the perinatal
     B **False**   mortality rate in diabetic pregnancy is higher than in
     C **True**   the overall population mainly due to congenital
     D **True**   malformation. The plaentas are usually big and are
     E **True**   not implicated in intrauterine death. Control of blood
                     sugar does reduce the incidence of fetal
                     abnormalities and macrosomia but does not
                     eliminate them. Medium and long term glucose
                     control is monitored by the level of glycosylated
                     haemoglobin less then 12%. Dexamethasone causes
                     a rise in blood sugar and insulin should be given
                     concurrently.

J M Brudenell in Ref 3 Vol 2

1.26 In assessing thyroid function in pregnancy the following tests are useful:
A   serum thyroxine (T₄)
B   free thyroxine index (FTI)
C   thyroid stimulating hormone (TSH)
D   protein bound iodine (PBI)
E   serum thyroxine binding globulin (TBG)

1.27 Anti thyroid drugs, such as carbimazole, used in the treatment of thyrotoxicosis in pregnancy
A   should be given in large doses to maintain a slightly hypothyroid state
B   cross the placenta
C   should be given initially with propanolol if symptoms are severe
D   cause tremor and palpations
E   are secreted in significant quantities in breast milk

1.28 Maternal rubella infection in early pregnancy
A   was first reported as harmful from Australia
B   is characterized by a vesicular rash
C   is teratogenic in 100% of cases before ten weeks gestation
D   is characterized by sub-occipital lymphadenopathy
E   causes patent ductus arteriosus in the fetus

1.29 The effects of intra-uterine rubella infection include
A   blindness
B   deafness
C   Hutchinsons teeth
D   intra-uterine growth retardation
E   hepatosplenomegaly.

(*Answers overleaf*)

1.26 A **False**   On account of the increase of thyroid binding protein
     B **True**   stimulated by oestrogens neither total serum
     C **True**   thyroxine or PBI are reliable indicators of thyroid
     D **False**   function in pregnancy. The FTI corrects for this
     E **False**   variable and is useful, whilst the TSH also reflects
                     thyroid function being reduced by a negative
                     feedback mechanism.

D A D Montgomery and J M G Harley in Ref 5

1.27 A **False**   Carbimazole should be given in the smallest dose
     B **True**   possible to control symptoms and if control is
     C **True**   difficult a slightly hyperthyroid state is preferable. It
     D **False**   is sometimes used in conjunction with thyroxine.
     E **True**   Transplacental passage is minimized by low dosage,
                     but passage into breast milk occurs and breast
                     feeding is contra indicated. Tremor and palpitations
                     are more likely to be due to poor control of
                     symptoms rather than a side effect of the drug.

D A D Montgomery & J M G Harley in Ref 5

1.28 A **True**   The harmful effects of maternal rubella infection
     B **False**   were first reported from Australia by Gregg. The type
     C **False**   of defect depends upon susceptibility and period of
     D **True**   gestation but the earlier it occurs the more serious is
     E **True**   the teratogenic effect. Many cardiac lesions occur but
                     patent ductus arteriosus is the most common.
                     Rubella is characterized by a maculopapular rash and
                     lymph node enlargement typically in the posterior
                     cervical area.

D Harvey & I Kovar in Ref 3 Vol 1

1.29 A **True**   The effects of intra-uterine rubella depend on the
     B **True**   period of gestation. Teratogenesis occurs with infection
     C **False**   before ten weeks' gestation and this includes
     D **True**   congenital defects of the heart and great vessels,
     E **True**   cataracts, microcephaly, deafness and
                     thrombocytopaenic purpura. Even in late pregnancy
                     serious defects include deafness, mental retardation,
                     intrauterine growth retardation and liver damage.

D Harvey & I Kovar in Ref 3 Vol 1

1.30 The following hormones in the fetal circulation are predominantly of maternal origin:
A   oestrogens
B   insulin
C   adrenocorticotrophic hormone
D   progesterone
E   thyroid stimulating hormone

1.31 The following drugs are known to adversely affect the fetus when prescribed during pregnancy:
A   Thiazide diuretics
B   Tetracyclines
C   Metronidazole
D   Heparin
E   Azathioprine

1.32 Chronic rheumatic heart disease in pregnancy
A   is becoming more common
B   should be treated with Digoxin
C   should have prophylactic antibiotics during pregnancy
D   is characterised by an irregular pulse
E   is an indication for Caesarean section

1.33 Phaeochromocytoma complicating pregnancy
A   is characteristically associated with paroxysmal hypertension
B   is associated with increased urinary excretion of hydroxyindole acetic acid (HIAA)
C   is usually sited in the adrenal cortex
D   causes obstetric collapse
E   is associated with glucose intolerance

(*Answers overleaf*)

1.30 A **True** Maternal sex steroid hormones predominate in the
    B **False** fetal circulation, with neonatal breast enlargement
    C **False** and menstruation being a feature of their withdrawal.
    D **True** Glucose does cross the placenta but the fetus
    E **False** synthesizes its own insulin which may become
excessive in a diabetic patient, because of fetal
hyperglycaemia. Pituitary trophic hormones are too
large to cross the placenta and the fetus controls its
own thyroid and adrenocortical function.

Ref 4

1.31 A **True** Thiazide diuretics are rarely indicated during
    B **True** pregnancy and cause thrombocytopaenia and
    C **False** bleeding disorders in the neonate. Heparin, not
    D **False** crossing the placenta, is the drug of choice for
    E **False** anti-coagulation. Although an immunosuppressant
and potentially toxic, experience of Azathioprine in
chronic auto immune diseases and renal transplant
patients has as yet shown no adverse effect.
Metronidazole is safe in low dosage but Tetracyclines
produce staining of primary and secondary dentition.

S Wood & L Beeley in Ref 5

1.32 A **False** On account of the reduced incidence of acute
    B **False** rheumatic fever, chronic rheumatic heart disease has
    C **False** become less common. Only when it is complicated
    D **False** should digoxin be used and young patients rarely
    E **False** have dysrhythmias, although atrial fibrillation may
occur. Unless there is additional obstetric
complication Caesarean section is not indicated and
antibiotics are only required to cover delivery.

P Szekely & L Snaith in Ref 5

1.33 A **True** The hypertension associated with
    B **False** phaechromacytoma is characteristically paroxysmal
    C **True** and the patient may be normotensive when first
    D **True** seen. It is a tumour of the adrenal medulla, usually
    E **True** single and on the right side. It may also be situated
anywhere along the sympathetic chain. It is often
diagnosed at post mortem and obstetric collapse
may occur due to haemorrhage into the tumour on
account of mechanical factors at delivery cutting off
the hormone excretion. Phaeochromocytomas
secrete adrenaline and noradrenaline which appear
in the urine as vanillyl mandelic acid (VMA). Blood
sugar is often raised due to the increased adrenaline.

D A D Montgomery and J M G Harley in Ref 5

1.34 A diagnosis of pre eclampsia in a patient at thirty-seven weeks gestation with a blood pressure of 160/100 mm mercury would be supported by
  A   mild ankle swelling
  B   proteinuria of 3 g per day
  C   a blood pressure at 16 weeks gestation of 160/100 mm Hg
  D   epigastric pain
  E   a parity of four

1.35 A 30-year-old multigravid patient with proteinuria and hypertension at 32 weeks gestation
  A   probably has pre eclampsia
  B   on optic fundal examination will have new vessel formation
  C   should have a 24-hour urine collection for vanillyl mandelic acid
  D   should be treated with long-term Hydralazine
  E   will not show characteristic pathological placental changes

1.36 Proteinuria in pre-eclampsia
  A   is usually tubular
  B   is associated with hyperlipidaemia
  C   is poorly selective
  D   contains IgG
  E   may produce the nephrotic syndrome

1.37 Theories of the pathogenesis of pre eclampsia include immune complex formation. The following statements are correct:
  A   trophoblastic antigens cross-react with glomerular basement membrane antigens
  B   trophoblastic antigenic stimulus is weak
  C   there is increased circulating level of Immuno globulin G in pre eclampsia
  D   there is an elevation of anti HLA antibodies in pre eclampsia
  E   immunofluorescence studies show immumoglobulin deposition in kidneys

1.38 The aetiology of pre-eclampsia is obscure, but which of the following statements are correct:
  A   disseminated intramuscular coagulation probably has a causative role in pre-eclampsia
  B   heparin may improve the clinical course of the disease
  C   hypertensive primigravidae have a lower renin than normotensive controls
  D   pre-eclamptics have increased vaso-responsiveness to infused angiotensin II
  E   a reduced maternal immune response is an important factor in the aetiology of pre-eclampsia

(Answers overleaf)

1.34 A **False**   Mild ankle oedema occurs in more than 50% of
     B **True**   normal pregnancies and is not helpful. A proteinuria
     C **False**   of 3 g per day is significant and is almost certainly
     D **True**   due to pre eclampsia at this stage of gestation. If the
     E **False**   blood pressure was raised in the first trimester, then
                   there is chronic hypertension. Pre eclampsia is less
                   common in multiparous patients and it may cause
                   visual disturbance, headaches or epigastric pain.

1.35 A **False**   Pre eclampsia is essentially a disease of
     B **False**   primigravidae and hypertension in multigravid
     C **True**   patients is more likely to be renal or essential in
     D **False**   origin. Fatalities in pregnancy occur with
     E **True**   undiagnosed phaeochromocytoma and VMA assays
                   should be performed. There are no characteristic
                   changes in the placenta and new vessel formation
                   will not be found in the optic fundus. New vessel
                   formation is characteristic of diabetic retinopathy, not
                   hypertensive retinopathy.

1.36 A **False**   The proteinuria of pre-eclampsia occurs from defects
     B **True**   in the basement membrane and is glomerular and
     C **True**   nearly always poorly selective, i.e. large molecules
     D **True**   (IgG and larger) pass through into the glomerular
     E **True**   filtrate. If heavy, i.e. more than 5 g/day the
                   proteinuria may produce profound
                   hypoalbuminaemia, hyperlipidaemia and oedema
                   identical to that found in the nephrotic syndrome.

J W W Studd in Ref 5

1.37 A **True**   Trophoblastic antigens are weak and cross-react with
     B **True**   glomerular basement membrane. Pre eclampsia does
     C **False**   have certain similarities to 'allergic nephritis' with
     D **False**   deposition of immunoglobulin G, immunoglobulin
     E **True**   M, and complement as well as fibrin in the basement
                   membrane. There is decreased immunoglobulin G
                   and decreased HLA antibodies suggesting a reduced
                   maternal immune response to the fetoplacental
                   homograft.

O Petrucco in Ref 3 Vol 1

1.38 A **False**   Disseminated intravascular coagulation occurs in
     B **False**   pre-eclampsia but is probably not causative and
     C **True**   removal of the coagulopathy by heparin does not
     D **True**   improve the condition. Hypertensive patients have a
     E **True**   decreased plasma renin and angiotensin, but have an
                   exaggerated vascular response to infused
                   angiotensin II.

O Petrucco in Ref 3 Vol 1

1.39 The pathological features of the renal changes associated with pre eclampsia include
    A increased glomerular filtration rate
    B increase in mesangial cells and matrix
    C fibrinoid necrosis of glomerular arterioles
    D fibrin-like deposits in the glomeruli
    E lymphocytic infiltration of the proximal convoluted tubule

1.40 Ec lampsia
    A occurs more commonly at high altitude
    B should be treated by intravenous diuretics
    C causes respiratory failure
    D causes hyperpyrexia
    E causes oliguria with a urinary urea to plasma urea ratio of greater than 10

1.41 Preterm labour
    A is defined in Britain as any labour commencing before 37 completed weeks from conception
    B is the leading cause of perinatal mortality in Britain
    C has a lower limit of 28 weeks' gestation
    D is more common in patients with a pelvic kidney
    E tends to recur in subsequent pregnancies

1.42 Twin pregnancy occurs
    A in 1:120 pregnancies in Britain
    B more commonly in black patients
    C less commonly in Japan than in Europe
    D more frequently in patients being treated with bromocriptine for infertility
    E more commonly in older patients

(*Answers overleaf*)

1.39 A **False**   Renal biopsies performed in pre eclampsia have
      B **True**   shown characteristic reversible features mainly in the
      C **False**   glomeruli. Afferent glomerular arterioles are
      D **True**   narrowed with a reduction in blood flow and
      E **False**   glomerular filtration rate. There is swelling of
                     capillary endothelial cells, increase in mesangial cells
                     and matrix and granular fibrin like deposition within
                     endothelial cells, in the mesangial matrix and in
                     continuity with basement membrane.

C J Dewhurst in Ref 4

1.40 A **False**   Eclampsia occurs more commonly in coastal regions
      B **False**   and should be treated by anti-convulsants, possibly
      C **True**   with anti-hypertensives. Hypovolaemia already exists
      D **True**   and diuretics should not be given. Complications
      E **True**   include cerebral haemorrhage, renal failure and
                     inhalation pneumonia. Oliguria may be pre-renal
                     with a concentrated urine and a high urinary urea to
                     plasma urea ratio. It may also be due to acute tubular
                     or cortical necrosis with a low urinary urea to plasma
                     urea ratio which has a worse prognosis and may
                     require renal dialysis.

J W W Studd in Ref 7

1.41 A **False**   Preterm labour is defined in Britain as any labour
      B **True**   commencing before 37 completed weeks have
      C **False**   elapsed from the last menstrual period. In about 50%
      D **True**   of perinatal deaths prematurity is a factor. There is no
      E **True**   lower limit of gestation or birth weight. Because of
                     the association of renal tract abnormalities with
                     uterine abnormalities preterm labour in more
                     common in such cases. Previous preterm delivery is
                     the most important predictive factor for subsequent
                     pregnancies.

Ref 8

1.42 A **False**   Twin pregnancy occurs in about 1:80 pregnancies in
      B **True**   Britain. It is commoner in black races (1:30) and
      C **True**   much less common in Japan (1:200). While multiple
      D **False**   pregnancy occurs more commonly in infertile
      E **True**   patients treated with clomiphene or pergonal this is
                     not the case with bromocriptine, which acts by
                     restoring normal ovulation. Dizygotic twin pregnancy
                     is commoner in parous patients as well as in older
                     patients.

Ref 9

1.43 Twin pregnancy shows an increase in the following complication:
A Placental abruption
B Pre eclampsia
C Oligohydramnios
D Polycythaemia
E Post partum haemorrhage

1.44 Dizygotic twins
A are more common following ovulation induction
B are more common than monozygotic twins
C are complicated by the twin transfusion syndrome
D should be monitored during pregnancy by urinary oestriols
E are more common in thin women

1.45 The following neurological disorders are recognized complications of pregnancy:
A diplopia
B Bell's palsy
C nystagmus
D carpal tunnel syndrome
E meralgia paraesthetica

1.46 The following are characteristic skin manifestations of normal pregnancy:
A palmar erythema
B pemphigoid
C vitiligo
D spider naevi
E chloasma

1.47 Auscultatory findings in a normal pregnant woman characteristically include
A a short diastolic murmur at the apex
B a bruit over the renal angles
C an ejection systolic murmur over the base of the heart
D a third heart sound
E an ejection click

(*Answers overleaf*)

1.43 A **True**   Twin pregnancy is associated with an increase in
     B **True**   almost every pregnancy complication. All types of
     C **False**   haemorrhage are more common, as is pre
     D **False**   eclampsia; polyhydramnios and anaemia due to
     E **True**   increased demand of iron and folic acid are also
                    common.

Ref 9

1.44 A **True**   Dizygotic (non-identical) twins are more common in
     B **True**   older women and after induction of ovulation. There
     C **False**   is the suggestion that they may be more common in
     D **False**   fat women and they are certainly more frequent than
     E **False**   monozygotic twins. The twin transfusion syndrome
                    occurs in monozygotic twins. The standard
                    biochemical placental function tests are
                    inappropriate for monitoring twin pregnancy as one
                    twin may be distressed or dead, with increasing total
                    hormone outputs.

Ref 9

1.45 A **False**   Bell's palsy, carpal tunnel syndrome and meralgia
     B **True**   paraesthetica are nerve compression syndromes
     C **False**   probably due to changes in body fluid distribution
     D **True**   which regress after the delivery. Diplopia and
     E **True**   nystagmus may be features of serious neurological
                    disease and should lead to further investigation.

Ref 10

1.46 A **True**   There are numerous physiological changes affecting
     B **False**   the skin in pregnancy, which include palmar
     C **False**   erythema, spider naevi and chloasma. All three are
     D **True**   probably related to elevated oestrogen levels,
     E **True**   regressing soon after delivery in the majority of
                    cases. Palmar erythema and spider naevi are also
                    seen in non pregnant patients with chronic liver
                    disease who cannot metabolize and excrete
                    oestrogens. Pemphigoid and vitiligo are unrelated to
                    pregnancy.

Ref 10

1.47 A **False**   The hyperkinetic circulatory state of normal
     B **False**   pregnancy is manifested by a full pulse, a forceful
     C **True**   cardiac impulse, an ejection systolic murmur
     D **True**   probably from the pulmonary artery and a third heart
     E **False**   sound. In the absence of other features suggestive of
                    heart disease, these are benign. Any diastolic
                    murmur suggests a pathological cause and a bruit
                    over the renal angles suggests renal artery stenosis,
                    being of special significance in a hypertensive patient.

Ref 10

1.48 The folowing haematological indices would be considered normal in the second half of the normal pregnancy:
A   Mean cell volume (MCV) 105 femtolitres
B   Erythrocyte sedimentation rate (ESR) 50 mm per hour
C   Platelet count of 100 000 per ml
D   White cell count (WCC) 12×10^9/l
E   Reticulocyte count 15% of red cells

1.49 Chronic glomerulonephritis associated with pregnancy
A   is treated with steroids
B   is associated with a worse fetal outcome even if normotensive
C   leads to permanent deterioration in renal function
D   presents as the nephrotic syndrome
E   is often caused by Escherichia coli

1.50 The following statements concerning gastro-intestinal problems in pregnancy are correct:
A   Infertility is commoner in patients with Crohn's disease
B   Ulcerative colitis originating during pregnancy has a bad prognosis
C   Peptic ulceration becomes more troublesome during pregnancy
D   Intestinal obstruction is a recognised complication in ileostomy patients
E   Untreated coeliac disease carries an increased risk of spontaneous abortion.

1.51 In ante partum pre-eclampsia (pregnancy induced hypertension)
A   treatment with diuretics is beneficial.
B   primary treatment with intravenous Diazoxide is contra-indicated.
C   plasma magnesium levels should be kept at approximately 20 mEq/L during magnesium sulphate therapy.
D   maternal placental blood flow falls less than 50% of normal.
E   there is a greater incidence of hypertension in later life.

(*Answers overleaf*)

1.48 A **False**   The ESR and WCC are frequently elevated in normal
      B **True**   pregnancy and are not sensitive indicators of
      C **False**   disease. White cell count is especially elevated in
      D **True**   labour, rising to $20 \times 10^9/l$ or above and often
      E **False**   leads to a futile search for infection when associated
                      with a slightly raised body temperature. MCV of 105
                      femtolitres indicates large red cells — a macrocytosis
                      — which is pathological. A platelet count of 100 000
                      per ml is abnormally low and a reticulocyte count
                      should not be higher than 2%.

Ref 10

1.49 A **False**   The different types of glomerulonephritis are thought
      B **False**   to be immunologically mediated and are not infective
      C **False**   in origin. Some cases of acute glomerulonephritis are
      D **True**   treated with steroids. Renal function does not
      E **False**   deteriorate due to pregnancy, but if hypertension is
                      severe and gross oedema and proteinuria develop,
                      then fetal outcome is compromised.

Ref. 10

1.50 A **True**   Crohn's disease may produce peritubal adhesions
      B **True**   and hence infertility. Dyspareunia and reduced
      C **False**   frequency of intercourse is also likely if there is large
      D **True**   bowel disease. Ulcerative colitis originating during
      E **True**   pregnancy often deteriorates, but gastric and
                      duodenal ulcer usually improve. Ileostomy patients
                      often have uneventful normal vaginal delivery but
                      intestinal obstruction from adhesions is a serious
                      risk. Untreated coeliac disease predisposes to
                      spontaneous abortion.

J P Miller in Ref. 5 Vol. 4 No. 2

1.51 A **False**   Diuretic therapy is of no value and is probably contra
      B **True**   indicated in pre-eclampsia. Diazoxide may cause
      C **False**   profound hypotension and fetal death. Magnesium
      D **True**   sulphate is a simple safe and effective therapy which
      E **True**   is rarely used in the United Kingdom. It is necessary
                      to monitor toxicity by tendon reflexes and by
                      maintaining plasma levels below 7 mEq/L. Although
                      hypertension is more common in later life this does
                      not imply that pre-eclampsia causes this long-term
                      problem.

Ref 11

1.52 A previously fit 32 year old primigravida at 28 weeks' gestation presents with intractable itching and jaundice. She is otherwise well. There is no hepatomegaly. The serum bilirubin is 80 μmol/l (5 mg/100 ml), the alkaline phosphatase elevated and the gamma glutamyl transpeptidase elevated.
A the most probable diagnosis is viral hepatitis
B delivery is indicated
C acute fatty liver is a probable sequel
D cholestyramine should be prescribed
E the subsequent use of oral contraceptives should be discouraged

1.53 The following are characteristic features of acute fatty liver of pregnancy:
A abdominal pain
B headache
C uraemia
D periportal fat deposition on liver biopsy
E fatty infiltration of the renal tubules

1.54 Acute appendicitis complicating pregnancy
A is less common than in the non-pregnant woman
B should be operated upon through a low paramedian incision
C is treated by appendicectomy and coincident Caesarean section if the fetus is mature
D mimics urinary tract infection
E is less common in black patients

1.55 Epileptic patients
A if controlled with Phenytoin have no increased risk of fetal abnormalities
B often require increased dosage of anti-convulsants during pregnancy
C if receiving Phenytoin therapy, may have an associated macrocytic blood picture with normal serum folate and B12
D should have barbiturates as a treatment of choice during pregnancy
E if receiving barbiturates, the babies are more likely to suffer from neonatal jaundice

(*Answers overleaf*)

1.52 A **False**   A previously fit pregnant patient with little
     B **False**   constitutional upset but complaining of pruritis and
     C **False**   jaundice at 28 weeks' gestation almost certainly has
     D **True**   intrahepatic cholestasis of pregnancy. Delivery is not
     E **True**   indicated and acute fatty liver is not associated with
                     this condition. Cholestyramine may relieve the
                     itching and possibly improve the fetal outcome.
                     Contraceptives are contraindicated as the pathology
                     depends upon their oestrogenic stimulus.

J P Miller in Ref 5

1.53 A **True**   Patients with this syndrome previously termed 'acute
     B **True**   yellow atrophy' present with abdominal pain,
     C **True**   vomiting and headaches. Jaundice and uraemia
     D **False**   occur. Centrilobular far deposition is seen on liver
     E **True**   biopsy and fatty infiltration of the renal tubules also
                     occurs. The maternal and perinatal outcome is poor.

J P Miller in Ref 5

1.54 A **True**   Acute appendicitis complicating pregnancy is often
     B **False**   diagnosed late because of its atypical features and its
     C **False**   comparative infrequency. The incision must be
     D **True**   paramedian over the point of maximum tenderness,
     E **True**   which may well be in the upper quadrant of the
                     abdomen in late pregnancy. The main differential
                     diagnosis is between urinary tract infection,
                     concealed antepartum haemorrhage and
                     appendicitis. Microscopy of the urine specimen is
                     essential. Appendicitis is less common in black
                     patients, although with changes in nutritional habits
                     and with urbanisation, this may not remain true.

1.55 A **False**   Both Phenytoin and barbiturates have been
     B **True**   incriminated in causing fetal abnormalities, but
     C **True**   changing from Phenytoin the most commonly
     D **False**   prescribed anti-convulsant during pregnancy, may
     E **False**   lead to loss of control and consequent morbidity.
                     Ideally, the anti-convulsant therapy should be
                     modified if necessary before a planned pregnancy.
                     Barbiturates induce liver enzymes and may well
                     reduce neonatal jaundice in premature neonates.

A Hopkins in Ref 5

1.56 Myasthenia gravis complicating pregnancy
A   is treated with anticholinesterase drugs
B   is an indication for elective Caesarean section
C   is associated with neonatal myasthenia
D   is most likely to deteriorate in the third trimester
E   is associated with a slow first stage of labour

1.57 Herpes gestationis
A   is caused by herpes virus
B   recurs in subsequent pregnancies
C   causes a bullous skin eruption
D   is treated with steroids
E   improves with plasmapheresis

1.58 An abdomino-pelvic X-ray of a pregnant woman
A   carries a risk to the fetus
B   is more reliable at detemining congenital abnormalities than ultrasonic scan
C   usually shows ossification of the upper tibial epiphysis at thirty nine weeks gestation
D   showing placental calcification confirms postmaturity
E   provides an assessment of placenta praevia

1.59 In the diagnosis of deep venous thrombosis in veins below the knee
A   the observation of calf pain, ankle swelling and localized tenderness will lead to a false positive diagnosis in about half the patients
B   about half the patients may have none of the above signs, but definite thrombosis
C   radioactive fibrinogen test is helpful in pregnancy
D   X-ray venography is contra-indicated in pregnancy
E   Homan's sign is diagnostic

(Answers overleaf)

1.56 A **True**   Myasthenia gravis is a disorder of motor end plate
     B **False**   function improved by increasing the amount of
     C **True**   transmitter substance acetylcholine. It is most likely
     D **False**   to deteriorate in the puerperium and is not an
     E **False**   indication for elective Caesarean section unless other
                    obstetric complications are present. Neonatal
                    myasthenia occurs in about 10% of cases. Uterine
                    muscle activity is unaffected and the first stage of
                    labour proceeds normally.

Ref 4

1.57 A **False**   Herpes gestationis is a bullous eruption in pregnancy
     B **True**   clinically similar to other herpetic lesions but not
     C **True**   caused by herpes virus. It is an auto immune disease
     D **True**   improved by steroids or plasmapheresis, but recurs
     E **True**   in subsequent pregnancies.

Ref 4

1.58 A **True**   X-ray of the fetus carries a much smaller risk of later
     B **False**   chidhood malignancy than originally thought, but it
     C **True**   does exist. X-rays will only show gross structural
     D **False**   abnormalities of the fetus and ultrasonic examination
     E **False**   is a better test. Ossification of the upper tibial
                    epiphysis usually occurs at thirty eight weeks
                    gestation although it is variable. X-ray assessment of
                    placenta praevia is difficult and unreliable.
                    Calcification of the placenta may be seen at any
                    gestation.

Ref 7

1.59 A **True**   Because the first two statements are true reliable
     B **True**   diagnostic tests are essential before commiting a
     C **False**   patient to the risk of anti-coagulant therapy. The I[131]
     D **False**   fibrinogen test is contra-indicated in pregnancy
     E **False**   because the isotope circulates systemically, X-ray
                    venograph below the knee using lead shielding to the
                    abdomen carries no risk. Homan's sign, along with
                    the other clinical observations, is not diagnostic.

P J Howie in Ref 5

1.60 The incidence of thrombo-embolism during pregnancy is increased in
A patients with nephrotic syndrome
B patients sterilized in the puerperium
C teenage pregnancies
D patients admitted to hospital during the antenatal period for reasons other than thrombosis
E pre-eclampsia

1.61 The syndrome of water intoxication associated with the use of large volumes of hypotonic fluid and oxytocin
A includes pulmonary oedema
B is manifested by loss of consciousness and fits
C is avoidable if blood electrolytes are checked after each litre of fluid given intravenously
D should be corrected by rapid infusion of hypertonic sodium chloride intravenously
E causes severe hypertension

1.62 The following are characteristic findings in pulmonary embolism:
A high PCO_2
B pH below 7.4
C abnormal ventilation lung scan
D raised serum Hydroxybutyrate Dehydrogenase (SHBD)
E $S_1 Q_{111} T_{111}$ pattern on electrocardiogram

1.63 Plasma potassium concentration
A accounts for more potassium than intracellular potassium.
B if grossly elevated will cause peaked T waves on electrocardiography.
C is reduced in Conn's syndrome.
D tends to be low in renal failure.
E should be maintained by supplements during prolonged intravenous therapy.

(*Answers overleaf*)

1.60 A **True**   Older patients, those having had an operative
     B **True**   delivery and those admitted to hospital during the
     C **False**   antenatal period, especially with hypertensive
     D **True**   disorders all have an increased risk of
     E **True**   thrombo-embolism. The common factor may be bed
                   rest. A feature of the nephrotic syndrome is a
                   thrombotic tendency. Oestrogens are
                   contra-indicated for suppression of lactation and
                   bromocriptine is an effective alternative although
                   breast support and analgesia is usually sufficient.

P W Howie in Ref 5

1.61 A **False**   This syndrome which is avoidable if blood
     B **True**   biochemistry is adequately monitored causes
     C **True**   cerebral symptoms because of entry of water into the
     D **False**   cells. The water does not remain extra-cellular;
     E **False**   oedema and hypertension are not prominent
                   features. Simply stopping oxytocin and the hypotonic
                   fluids leads to improvement. Gradual infusion of 5%
                   saline is the correct management as rapid infusion
                   may lead to dangerous swings of osmolality.

P Sanderson in Ref 13

1.62 A **False**   Patients with a pulmonary embolism are hypoxic
     B **False**   which leads to hyperventilation, a blowing off of CO_2
     C **False**   and a respiratory alkalosis. There is normal
     D **True**   ventilation but a perfusion scan will demonstrate the
     E **True**   area of embolus. A raised SHBD is the only
                   characteristic enzyme change and the usual ECG
                   change is of acute right heart strain, but the rare
                   finding of $S_1 Q_{111} T_{111}$ pattern is diagnostic of major
                   pulmonary embolism.

G Sutton in Ref 13

1.63 A **False**   Most potassium in the body is intracellular and
     B **True**   plasma potassium is a poor guide to the total body
     C **True**   potassium. Elevated levels of this ion cause peaking
     D **False**   of the T waves on the electrocardiogram. Metabolic
     E **True**   disturbances especially renal failure cause potassium
                   to be raised. A rare cause of depressed potassium
                   levels in Conn's syndrome which also causes
                   hypertension. The commonest cause of depressed
                   potassium is prolonged intravenous therapy. In these
                   circumstances electrolytes should be monitored and
                   supplements given.

P Sanderson in Ref 13

1.64 Women who have undergone renal transplantation
A have a conception rate equal to those on haemodialysis for chronic renal failure
B have an increased incidence of fetal abnormality due to azothiaprine
C should be monitored for rejection episodes during pregnancy
D are usually delivered by Caesarean section
E have an increased incidence of intra uterine growth retardation

1.65 Reversible pre-renal failure (as seen in the oliguric patient after a post partum haemorrhage) may be distinguished from established renal failure by the following findings:
A urine output of more than 10 ml/h
B the absence of oedema
C a urine osmolality of greater than 600 mmol/kg
D urinary sodium of less than 10 mmol/l
E a high urine to plasma ratio of urea (> 7:1)

1.66 The following features seen on microscopic examination of a fresh specimen of urine from a normal female are clearly abnormal:
A squamous epithelial cells
B hyaline casts
C densely granular casts
D cystine crystals
E red cell casts

1.67 Renal glomerular function may be accurately assessed by the following measurements:
A plasma urate
B plasma bicarbonate
C plasma urea
D urinary concentrating ability
E creatinine clearance

1.68 The following are known to cause acute renal failure:
A malaria
B sickle cell trait
C septicaemia
D concealed antepartum haemorrhage
E systemic lupus erythematosus

(Answers overleaf)

1.64 A **False**   Patients on haemodialysis rarely conceive and often
      B **False**   abort, but patients who have received a transplant
      C **True**   often have successful pregnancies. The
      D **False**   immunosuppressant azothiaprine is not associated
      E **True**   with fetal abnormalities. Although the kidney is
                      positioned in the iliac fossa vaginal delivery is to be
                      preferred and presents no problem. Hypertension is
                      often a feature and associated with fetal growth
                      retardation.

S M Wood & J D Blainey in Ref 5

1.65 A **False**   Most patients with renal failure of any type are
      B **False**   oliguric or anuric and patients in acute renal failure
      C **True**   do not have oedema. Pre-renal failure is
      D **True**   characterized by the kidney maintaining its ability to
      E **True**   concentrate urine, conserve sodium and excrete
                      urea. The urinary osmolality is usually greater than
                      600 mmol/kg, urinary sodium less than 10 mmol/l
                      and urinary urea much greater than plasma urea.
                      Progressive failure results in changes in these values
                      and may be avoided by aggressive treatment,
                      especially by volume replacement in the pre-renal
                      phase.

A R Clarkson in Ref 13

1.66 A **False**   Squamous epithelial cells are seen frequently in such
      B **False**   specimens and are contaminants from the vulva even
      C **True**   when good collection technique has been used.
      D **True**   Normal people may have hyaline casts in the urine
      E **True**   but granular casts suggest nephritis. Red cell casts
                      suggest glomerular bleeding and cystine crystals
                      occur in homozygous cystinurics.

D N S Kerr in Ref 13

1.67 A **False**   Although all of the above measurements may be
      B **False**   abnormal in renal disease only the creatinine
      C **False**   clearance provides an accurate method of assessing
      D **False**   glomerular function. The plasma urea is affected by
      E **True**   other variables and is not specific. Urine
                      concentrating ability reflects renal tubular function.

D N S Kerr in Ref 13

1.68 A **True**   Careful monitoring of renal function is necessary in
      B **False**   eclampsia, septicaemia and hypovolaemia to detect
      C **True**   the onset of renal failure. Rapid replacement of blood
      D **True**   volume after haemorrhage should avoid renal failure.
      E **True**   Primary renal diseases, various drugs and infusions
                      cause acute renal failure.

A R Clarkson in Ref 13

1.69 Pregnant patients with haemoglobinopathies
A   may have sickle disease with genotype SC
B   are less often iron deficient than controls
C   may have alpha thalassaemia major and severe anaemia
D   should be transfused in order to keep Haemoglobin S below 40%
E   who have sickle cell trait have unchanged perinatal mortality

1.70 Perinatal mortality rates are adversely affected by
A α thalassaemia minor
B   HbSS disease
C   beta thalassaemia minor
D   HbSC disease
E   sickle thalassaemia

1.71 β thalassaemia
A   if heterozygous causes severe anaemia
B   if homozygous is incompatible with life
C   occurs in black patients
D   manifests as haemolytic crises if heterozygous
E   can be diagnosed prenatally

1.72 Which of the following statements are true:
A   haemophilia is autosomal recessive
B   Huntington's chorea is autosomal dominant
C   Duchenne muscular dystrophy is sex-linked recessive
D   maple syrup urine disease is autosomal dominant
E   spina bifida is autosomal recessive

1.73 Idiopathic thrombocytopaenic purpura (ITP)
A   is associated with post partum haemorrhage
B   is associated with increased perinatal mortality
C   is confirmed by increased metamyelocytes in the bone marrow aspirate
D   is treated by splenectomy after pregnancy
E   is an auto immune disease

(*Answers overleaf*)

1.69 A **True**   Patients with sickle cell disease may be SS, SC or S
     B **False** thalassaemia but alpha thalassaemia major is
     C **False** incompatible with life (causing hydrops fetalis and
     D **True**   stillbirths). Haemoglobin S levels should be kept
     E **True**   below 40% by top up or by exchange transfusion.
                  Patients with haemoglobinopathies have iron
                  deficiency in the same frequency as found in the
                  general population. Sickle cell trait does not alter the
                  perinatal mortality.

S M Tuck & J White in Ref 3 Vol 1

1.70 A **False** Sickle cell trait and the thalassaemia minor
     B **True**   conditions are benign disorders as far as perinatal
     C **False** and maternal mortality rates are concerned. HbSS
     D **True**   disease and HbSC disease however have much
     E **True**   increased fetal loss and indeed a significant maternal
                  mortality. Fetal loss in sickle thalassaemia is slightly
                  lower than in HbSS or HbSC disease.

S M Tuck & J White in Ref 3 Vol 1

1.71 A **False** β thalassaemia minor (heterozygous) may be
     B **False** asymptomatic and causes mild anaemia. The major
     C **True**   form (homozygous) is a crippling disorder with
     D **False** severe anaemia and death in childhood without
     E **True**   intensive treatment. Thalassaemia occurs mainly in
                  people of Mediterranean origin but should be
                  considered as a cause of refractory hypochromic
                  anaemia in any race. Prenatal diagnosis by fetoscopic
                  blood sampling is practised.

C R Whitfield in Ref 4

1.72 A **False** Haemophilia and Duchenne muscular dystrophy are
     B **True**   sex-linked recessive diseases appearing in males.
     C **True**   The inborn errors of metabolism are all autosomal
     D **False** recessive. Neural tube defects (apart from being
     E **False** more common in Celts) are not genetically
                  determined.

Ref 16

1.73 A **False** ITP, an auto immune disease, causes purpura during
     B **True**   pregnancy. Bleeding problems are unlikely unless the
     C **False** platelet count is below 50 000/mm^3. It is associated
     D **True**   with increased maternal and perinatal mortality and
     E **True**   is confirmed by finding increased megakaryocytes on
                  bone marrow aspirate and is treated by splenectomy.

C R Whitfield in Ref 4

1.74 The following are recommended for the prevention of Rh isoimmunisation:
A   Antenatal anti-D administration of 100 micrograms at 28 weeks and 34 weeks
B   100 micrograms of anti-D post partum
C   50 micrograms of anti-D following abortion
D   A Kleihauer test after delivery of all Rh negative patients
E   300 micrograms of anti-D at 28 weeks

1.75 Plasmapheresis has been used effectively in
A   rhesus disease
B   herpes gestationis
C   diabetes mellitus
D   sickle cell disease
E   recurrent abortion

1.76 Acute cortical necrosis characteristically follows
A   placental abruption
B   post partum haemorrhage
C   tissue damage
D   septic shock
E   road traffic accidents

1.77 The following statements about L/S ratios are correct:
A   true idiopathic respiratory distress syndrome does not occur when L/S ratio is greater than 2
B   results are affected by bloodstaining of amniotic fluid
C   results correlate well with the shake test
D   stressed fetuses may have no respiratory difficulty although the L/S ratio is much less than 2
E   the test is indicated in severe pre eclamptics

(*Answers overleaf*)

1.74 A **True**   A Kleihauer test is an obligatory investigation to
      B **True**   measure the volume of feto-maternal haemorrhage.
      C **True**   100 micrograms of anti-D given post partum would
      D **True**   only neutralize 4 ml of fetal blood in the maternal
      E **True**   serum and more may be necessary. Both regimens of
                      ante partum rhesus prophylaxis (A & E) are virtually
                      100% effective but the former is more economical. It
                      should be remembered that most 'failures' are due to
                      'administrative errors' and omission of anti-D
                      administration in patients at risk. This seems to be
                      particularly common after spontaneous abortion and
                      termination of pregnancy.

C R Whitfield in Ref 3

1.75 A **True**   Plasmapheresis is used in conditions where auto
      B **True**   antibody formation is a feature (auto immune
      C **False**   diseases). Removal of the plasma and separation of
      D **False**   the detrimental factor is possible but provides only
      E **False**   short term relief. It has been used effectively but has
                      limited clinical application in herpes gestationis and
                      rhesus disease when sensitisation has occurred.

Refs various

1.76 A **True**   Acute cortical necrosis is a most severe form of acute
      B **False**   renal failure which follows tissue damage, sepsis and
      C **True**   thromboplastin release. Placental abruption is oddly
      D **True**   enough similar to road traffic accidents in the
      E **True**   aetiology in that there is a vast amount of concealed
                      blood loss with tissue damage. Acute cortical necrosis
                      very rarely follows post partum haemorrhage, as this
                      produces hypovolaemia alone.

Ref 7

1.77 A **False**   Amniocentesis for the assessment of the L/S ratio is a
      B **True**   classic example of an over-used and abused
      C **True**   investigation with too many false positives or false
      D **True**   negatives to be of value except in the more extreme
      E **False**   dilemmas of diabetes or rhesus disease. RDS
                      certainly occurs when the L/S ratio is greater than 2.
                      Severe pre eclamptics need control of blood
                      pressure, delivery and intensive neonatal care. The
                      patient would usually be premature, the L/S ratio low
                      and irrelevant.

Ref 7

1.78 The following are associated with vomiting:
  A   ectopic pregnancy
  B   ulcerative colitis during pregnancy
  C   venous thrombosis during pregnancy
  D   missed abortion
  E   hydatidiform mole

1.79 The following statements about this diagram are correct

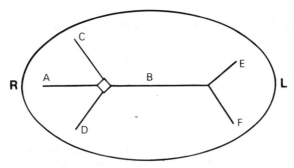

  A   E, F are the lamboidal sutures
  B   the point where B, E and F meet is the vertex
  C   moulding occurs at E, F — the occipital bone overlapping the
      parietal bones
  D   C, D is usually palpable in occipito-posterior positions
  E   this position is commonly found in an anthropoid pelvis

1.80 The normal umbilical cord
  A   contains two arteries
  B   contains Wharton's jelly
  C   pulsates at a rate equal to the maternal pulse rate
  D   is covered by amnion and chorion
  E   contains two veins

1.81 An anthropoid pelvis
  A   is associated with deep transverse arrest
  B   has a male-shaped brim
  C   is of good obstetric value
  D   has a narrow sub pubic arch
  E   is associated with spondylolisthesis

1.82 Placenta praevia
  A   is associated with an increased incidence of fetal abnormality
  B   is associated with an increased incidence of intrauterine
      growth retardation
  C   if anterior, is best treated by classical Caesarean section
  D   becomes symptomatic for the first time in labour in 15% of
      cases
  E   is more common in teenage pregnancy

(*Answers overleaf*)

1.78 A **True**   Ectopic pregnancy and especially hydatidiform mole
     B **False** are associated with vomiting, as in the normal
     C **False** pregnant state. Missed abortion is not associated
     D **False** with vomiting, probably because the hormone levels
     E **True**   have reverted to the non pregnant values.
                  Pyelonephritis is a common cause of vomiting.
                  Venous thrombosis is not associated with it.

Ref 4

1.79 A **True**   The vertex is the area bounded by the parietal
     B **False** eminences and the anterior and posterior fontanelles.
     C **False** The occipital bone is overlapped by the two parietal
     D **True**   bones with moulding. The head rarely engages in a
     E **False** transverse position with an anthropoid pelvis, as the
                  position is usually occipito-posterior and delivery
                  face to pubes.

Ref 6

1.80 A **True**   The normal umbilical cord contains two arteries and
     B **True**   one vein embedded in Wharton's jelly covered by
     C **False** amnion. The cord of an abnormal fetus may not
     D **False** show these characteristic features. As a part of the
     E **False** fetal circulation the cord pulsates at a rate equal to
                  the fetal heart rate.

Ref 6

1.81 A **False** An anthropoid pelvis has an oval brim and is
     B **False** associated with direct occipito-posterior position of
     C **True**   the fetal head. The head may descend through the
     D **False** pelvis which is of good obstetric value in this position
     E **False** and deliver face to pubes. It is the android pelvis
                  which is male-shaped, associated with oblique
                  posterior position, a narrow sub pubic arch and
                  complicated delivery. Spondylolisthesis which is the
                  displacement forwards of a lumbar vertebra, causes
                  narrowing of the true conjugate of the pelvic inlet.

Ref 6

1.82 A **True**   Placenta praevia is associated with an increased rate
     B **False** of fetal abnormalities, prematurity and breech
     C **False** presentation but not growth retardation. Given a
     D **True**   major degree of anterior placenta praevia a lower
     E **False** segment operation should still be performed.
                  Classical Caesarean section is very rarely performed
                  because of long term consequences.

Ref 6

1.83 In the treatment of a large concealed and revealed ante partum haemorrhage the following should be performed:
A   four-hourly vaginal examinations
B   measurement of plasma fibrinogen
C   early fluid replacement
D   blood gas measurement
E   delivery by Caesarean section if fetal heart present

1.84 A 20 year old primigravida is admitted with a painful antepartum haemorrhage. The blood pressure is 140/90 and the fetal heart is not heard. What treatment will she require:
A   syntocinon followed by amniotomy
B   blood replacement of approximately 2 units of blood
C   central venous catheterisation to measure pressure
D   epidural block
E   fresh frozen plasma transfusion before blood is available

1.85 Which of the following associations are correct:
A   William Hunter and the Gravid uterus
B   CHG Macafee and accidental haemorrhage
C   Elizabeth Nihill and pre-eclampsia
D   Charles White and puerperal sepsis
E   JW Ballantyne and antenatal care

1.86 The following methods of monitoring fetal wellbeing are of proven value:
A   oxytocin challenge test
B   urinary oestriols
C   plasma HPL
D   plasma heat stable alkaline phosphtase
E   kick counts

(*Answers overleaf*)

1.83 A **False**   The main maternal complications of a major ante
      B **True**   partum haemorrhage are renal failure due to
      C **True**   hypovolaemia and coagulation abnormalities.
      D **False**   Vaginal examination should be performed at least
      E **True**   two hours after amniotomy and syntocinon given if
                      there is no progress. The fetal heart is likely to be
                      absent, but if present early Caesarean section would
                      be performed by most obstetricians.

Ref 6

1.84 A **False**   This is a severe abruption with major concealed
      B **False**   blood loss causing pain and fetal death. She will
      C **True**   require urgent amniotomy followed by Syntocinon
      D **False**   within two hours if the cervix does not dilate. Note
      E **False**   that cervical dilatation may take place without
                      obvious contractions if the patient is in great pain.
                      Central venous pressure monitoring is vital as
                      vasospasm will make blood pressure an unreliable
                      indication of blood requirements. She will require in
                      excess of 4 units of blood transfusion. Normal saline
                      or dextran is adequate until blood is available.

1.85 A **True**   While not essential for examinations, the history of
      B **False**   obstetrics is fascinating. William Hunter published
      C **False**   his great anatomical atlas on the gravid uterus in
      D **True**   1774, Charles White of Manchester in 1773, made the
      E **True**   first significant advance in the understanding of
                      puerperal sepsis since Hippocrates, and J W
                      Ballantyne established the first antenatal clinic in the
                      early twentieth century. CHG Macafee demonstrated
                      the value of conservative management of placenta
                      praevia. Elizabeth Nihill was probably the most
                      famous midwife of the eighteenth century in that
                      she challenged the eminence of the male midwife
                      and of William Smellie in particular (1760). She
                      publicly and persistently criticized the use of forceps.

1.86 A **False**   Placental and fetal function tests come and go, with
      B **False**   most biochemical tests ultimately to be found
      C **False**   wanting. Currently the estimations of oestriols, HPL
      D **False**   and heat stable alkaline phosphatase have not
      E **True**   fulfilled their early promises. Oxytocin challenge
                      tests have never had support in this country but
                      cardiotocography (or non-stress test) in conjunction
                      with ultrasonic assessment of fetal growth are
                      valuable. Daily kick counts are certainly the cheapest
                      and might even be the best of these assessments of
                      fetal wellbeing.

1.87 The following compounds are prostaglandin synthetase inhibitors:
A mefenamic acid
B aspirin
C nifedepine
D naproxen
E indomethacin

1.88 Premature rupture of the membrane at thirty-two weeks gestation
A is associated with painful uterine contractions
B is associated with subsequent infertility
C is a contra-indication to digital examination of the cervical os
D is associated with fetal septicaemia
E should be confirmed by speculum examination

1.89 When a pre-term baby is delivered
A the nose should be aspirated before the oropharynx
B forceps should be used to protect the head
C it should be dried immediately
D a generous episiotomy is required
E a paediatrician must be present

1.90 The following tissues have a major role in initiation of labour at term:
A maternal pituitary gland
B fetal pituitary gland
C fetal adrenal gland
D intact maternal spinal cord
E fetal gonads

1.91 The onset of labour is encouraged by:
A prostaglandin F_2
B bound calcium ions
C progesterone
D oxytocin
E endoperoxides

(*Answers overleaf*)

1.87 A **True**   Non steroidal anti-inflammatory compounds
    B **True**   including mefenamic acid, aspirin, naproxen and
    C **False**   indomethacin have been studied because of their
    D **True**   action in inhibiting prostaglandin production. Clinical
    E **True**   application includes the treatment of
                 dysmenorrhoea, but their use in premature labour is
                 not approved because of their action in closing the
                 ductus arteriosus prematurely. Nifedepine is a
                 calcium antagonist which theoretically may depress
                 uterine activity.

Ref 8

1.88 A **False**   Premature membrane rupture by definition occurs
    B **True**   before the onset of painful uterine contractions and
    C **True**   may occur at any gestation. It should be confirmed
    D **True**   by speculum examination but digital examination is
    E **True**   forbidden because of the risk of chorioamnionitis,
                 intrauterine fetal infection and septicaemia. Bilateral
                 cornual blockage may follow this condition.

1.89 A **False**   The oropharynx should be aspirated before a nasal
    B **False**   stimulus produces a gasp and inhalation of
    C **True**   pharyngeal contents. Forceps do not protect the
    D **True**   premature skull and an episiotomy should be
    E **True**   adequate. Specialist paediatric cover should be
                 available and the maintenance of body temperature
                 is a priority.

Ref J K Ritchie & G McClure in Ref 3 Vol 2

1.90 A **False**   Secretion of trophic hormones by the fetal
    B **True**   hypothalamus and pituitary gland stimulates
    C **True**   secretion of cortisone by the adrenal cortex.
    D **False**   Subsequent events include a decrease in the level of
    E **False**   progesterone and consequent release of
                 prostaglandins.

B Schwartz in Ref 3 Vol 2

1.91 A **True**   Prostaglandin E_2, F_2, endoperoxides and
    B **False**   thromboxanes are thought to initiate the myometrial
    C **False**   contractions of normal labour and effect intracellular
    D **False**   AMP and free calcium ion. Oxytocin release is a
    E **True**   secondary change and may be relevant to the second
                 stage of labour while progesterone probably is active
                 in inhibiting uterine contractions.

B Schwartz in Ref 3 Vol 2

1.92 Oxytocin
A is a polypeptide hormone
B has an anti-diuretic hormone-like effect
C should be given at 0.2mu/minute to patients with prolonged labour
D causes water intoxication if given with large volumes of electrolyte free fluids
E is secreted by the anterior pituitary gland

1.93 The following statements about uterine activity are correct:
A Basal tone is highest in the periovulatory phase in the non pregnant uterus
B Pressures of 150 mmHg (20kPa) are developed in the second stage of labour
C Pressure is reliably quantified using external monitoring equipment
D It is affected by change of posture
E Cervical stretching induces stronger contractions

1.94 Epidural nerve block in labour
A involves the injection of an anaesthetic agent into the subarachnoid space
B causes transient hypotension
C increases the rate of forceps delivery
D increases the length of the first stage of labour
E is contra-indicated if the patient is on anti-coagulants

1.95 Ergometrine
A is given in a dose of 250–500 micrograms
B is combined with synthetic oxytocin in Syntometrine
C should not be given to a hypertensive patient
D acts within 60 seconds if given intravenously
E causes nausea and vomiting

(Answers overleaf)

1.92 A **True**   Oxytocin is a polypeptide hormone secreted by the
      B **True**   posterior pituitary gland and in its synthetic form is
      C **False**   called syntocinon. It should be given to treat
      D **True**   inefficient uterine action, but this is less common in
      E **False**   multiparous patients and mechanical obstruction
                        must be excluded; uterine rupture is a serious
                        potential complication. Oxytocin has an anti-diuretic
                        effect and when given with electrolyte-free fluid, such
                        as 5% Dextrose, it may cause water intoxication. The
                        normal dose for augmentation of labour is
                        2 mu/minute and subsequent incremental doses.

Ref 6

1.93 A **True**   The human uterus is active throughout life but the
      B **False**   pattern of activity varies. Various methods have been
      C **False**   used on a research basis to measure activity, but the
      D **True**   presence of a probe within the uterus is essential.
      E **True**   Turning a labouring patient on her side makes
                        contractions more intense but less frequent. Cervical
                        distension stimulates uterine activity temporarily
                        through the Ferguson reflex. The use of intra uterine
                        catheters has been associated with placental
                        damage, fetal distress and cord accidents.

J R Huey in Ref 5

1.94 A **False**   Injection is into the extradural space and a
      B **True**   sub-arachnoid injection may lead to serious side
      C **True**   effects. Hypotension is frequently observed after
      D **False**   epidural injection and should be corrected by an
      E **True**   intravenous infusion or prevented by pre-loading
                        with intravenous fluid. Many studies have shown the
                        rate of forceps deliveries to be increased, but there is
                        no evidence of prolongation of the first stage of
                        labour. Epidural injection is contra-indicated in a
                        patient on anti-coagulant therapy as an epidural
                        haematoma would be a serious complication.

J Selwyn-Crawford in Ref 3

1.95 A **True**   The recommended dose of ergometrine is 500
      B **True**   micrograms and it is combined with 5 units of
      C **True**   synthetic oxytocin in Syntometrine. Intravenously it
      D **True**   acts within sixty seconds but may especially then
      E **True**   cause nausea and vomiting. It should preferably not
                        be given to patients with a hypertensive tendency on
                        account of its vasopressor effect, but should
                        obviously not be withheld in cases of severe
                        haemorrhage.

Ref 6

1.96 The active management of labour includes the following characteristic features:
A induction of labour
B acceleration of labour
C use of a partogram
D a high Caesarean section rate
E continuous intrapartum fetal heart rate monitoring

1.97 Continuous intrapartum fetal heart rate monitoring
A has been responsible for a 25% decrease in perinatal mortality
B produces an overall increase in the Caesarean section rate
C should be used if possible in all patients in labour
D will reveal irregular fetal heart rate patterns in patients, 50% of whom will have fetal acidosis
E has decreased the risk of cerebral damage in high risk pregnancies

1.98 On admission in labour patients should have the following:
A bath
B phosphate enema
C vaginal examination
D amniotomy
E intravenous dextrose infusion

(*Answers overleaf*)

1.96 A **False**   The active management of labour as originally
     B **True**   described by O'Driscoll et al is applicable to
     C **True**   spontaneous primigravid labour. It involves selective
     D **False**   acceleration with syntocinon resulting in labours of
     E **True**   less than twelve hours duration and a low Caesarean
                    section rate. Partograms are essential for the graphic
                    recording of progress in labour and fetal heart rate
                    monitoring is necessary for what has become a high
                    risk labour.

L Cardozo, D M F Gibb & J W W Studd in Ref 3 Vol 2

1.97 A **False**   A difficult question and being controversial may be
     B **True**   best left unanswered. — (as you might lose marks for
     C **False**   being right!) Improvements in perinatal death rate
     D **True**   are as much due to changes in the management of
     E **False**   labour and changes in attitudes to forceps deliveries
                    as to monitoring. Three out of four control trials from
                    Sheffield, Denver and Melbourne have shown no
                    improvement in perinatal outcome in both high and
                    low risk groups when continuous fetal heart rate
                    monitoring is used. Monitoring also produces an
                    overall increase in Caesarean section rate which is
                    not as great if the monitoring is associated with fetal
                    blood sampling.

R J Parsons, V A Brown & I D Cooke in Ref 3 Vol 1

1.98 A **False**   Many traditional routine procedures are now being
     B **False**   questioned. These include the enema which probably
     C **True**   does not affect labour or decrease the incidence of
     D **False**   faecal soiling. A bath encourages ascending infection
     E **False**   and if anything, a shower is to be preferred. The full
                    pubic shave is also reprehensible. In high risk
                    pregnancies such time consuming procedures and
                    positively contra indicated; the enema in cases of
                    ruptured membranes with a preterm fetus is
                    especially dangerous. Correct management demands
                    an early vaginal examination, but amniotomy and
                    intravenous infusion should only be used when
                    indicated. Patients appreciate this sort of
                    consideration.

1.99 A head level of 'one fifth'
   A indicates that one fifth of the head is below the pelvic brim
   B indicates that the head is engaged
   C indicates that forceps may not be used
   D indicates that the head is at the level of the ischial spines
   E does not occur in a term brow presentation

**1.100 At the time of vaginal examination in labour the attendant
should**
   A catheterize the patient
   B wear a mask
   C drape the patient with sterile linen
   D use antiseptic cream
   E use sterile surgical gloves

**1.101 Which of the following statements about this primigravid
labour are correct:**

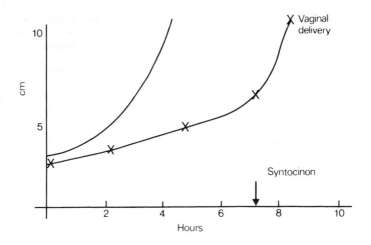

   A this patient has primary dysfunctional labour
   B syntocinon was given too late
   C there will be a 20% incidence of rotational forceps in this
patient
   D this patient probably has cephalo-pelvic disproportion
   E this patient should have continuous fetal heart rate
monitoring following acceleration of labour

(Answers overleaf)

1.99   A **False**   By convention, 'fifths' of head refer to the amount of
       B **True**   head palpable *above* the brim. One fifth above is
       C **False**   engaged, forceps and the ventouse may be used and
       D **False**   the abdominal levels bear little relationship to the
       E **True**   station estimated vaginally. The great advantage of
                      this classification is that the assessment of the head
                      yet to go through the pelvis is not confused by caput,
                      moulding and a varying depth of pelvis.

L D Cardozo, D M F Gibb & J W W Studd in Ref 3 Vol 2

1.100 A **False**   Vaginal examination should not become a clinical
       B **False**   surgical procedure. Draping and the use of masks
       C **False**   induces anxiety without adding to the safety of the
       D **True**   procedure. The examination requires an antiseptic
       E **False**   lubricant; sterile disposable gloves are adequate and
                      much cheaper. Catheterisation is unnecessary as a
                      routine procedure and may introduce infection.

1.101 A **True**   This patient has primary dysfunctional labour which
       B **True**   is most likely to be due to occipito-posterior position
       C **False**   or dysfunctional uterine action. Disproportion was
       D **False**   not present in this case, as the patient had a vaginal
       E **True**   delivery after augmentation of labour. The
                      Syntocinon was given late. As a high risk
                      dysfunctional labour the fetus needs continuous fetal
                      heart rate monitoring. The incidence of rotational
                      forceps will be higher than normal, but should be
                      much less than 20% even with an epidural.

L D Cardozo, D M F Gibb & J W W Studd in Ref 3 Vol 2

1.102 Which of the following statements about this labour are true:

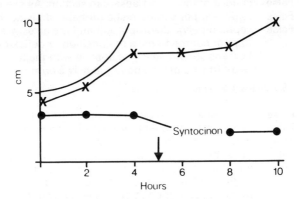

A   this patient has secondary arrest
B   this patient has had too many vaginal examinations
C   she has a 20% chance of a Caesarean section if a
    primigravida
D   she should have a trial of forceps in the operating theatre if
    the head is two-fifths above the brim
E   probably has cephalo-pelvic disproportion

1.103 Face presentation in labour
A   occurs in 1:1500 births
B   if mento-posterior, is favourable for a vaginal delivery
C   is associated with prematurity
D   results in the presentation of the sub-occipito-bregmatic
    diameter of the fetal head at the pelvic brim
E   is associated with anencephaly

1.104 The following statements about breech delivery are correct:
A   Lövset's manoeuvre is employed to deliver the head
B   breech extraction is less hazardous than assisted breech
    delivery
C   Wrigley's forceps are best suited for delivery of the
    after-coming head
D   the Mauriceau-Smellie-Veit method is used to deliver the
    after-coming head
E   fetal asphyxia is a more common cause of fetal death than
    intracranial haemorrhage

(*Answers overleaf*)

1.102 A **True**   This patient has secondary arrest which has
      B **False**   responded to Syntocinon. She has less than a 10%
      C **False**   chance of having a Caesarean section. As she is likely
      D **False**   to deliver per vaginam she probably does not have
      E **False**   cephalo-pelvic disproportion and the arrest was due
                     to poor contractions, a malposition or deflexion.
                     Forceps should never be applied with the head
                     two-fifths palpable above the pelvic brim.

L Cardozo, D M F Gibb & J W W Studd in Ref 3 Vol 2

1.103 A **False**   Face presentation occurs in about 1:500 labours
      B **False**   being associated with prematurity, anencephaly and
      C **True**   pelvic malformation. It results in the presentation of
      D **False**   the submento-vertical diameter at the pelvic brim
      E **True**   and if it rotates to a mento-anterior position then
                     vaginal delivery is likely. If it rotates to a
                     mento-posterior position it is less favourable and
                     Caesarean section may be necessary.

E D Morris in Ref 4

1.104 A **False**   Breech extraction carries a much higher fetal
      B **False**   mortality than assisted breech delivery and rough
      C **False**   handling of the trunk may lead to visceral damage.
      D **True**   Lövset's manoeuvre is used to deliver extended arms
      E **False**   and the Mauriceau-Smellie-Veit method may be used
                     to deliver the head. Wrigley's forceps are too small
                     for delivery after-coming head and long handled
                     forceps are more appropriate. Fetal death has been
                     shown to be more commonly due to intracranial
                     haemorrhage than fetal asphyxia and therefore slow,
                     careful, deliberate delivery is desirable.

N Duignan in Ref 3 Vol 2

1.105 Transverse lie of the fetus
    A should be treated by internal podalic version if the fetus is dead and the cervix fully dilated
    B may be treated by use of a Blond Heidler instrument
    C recurs in subsequent pregnancies
    D is associated with renal tract abnormalities
    E should be treated expectantly at 36 weeks' gestation

1.106 Preterm delivery
    A occurs in 12% of births in Britain
    B when associated with fetal or maternal disorders has a higher mortality than when spontaneous and uncomplicated
    C is reduced by the prophylactic use of beta mimetic drugs
    D is associated with Asherman's syndrome
    E is reduced in incidence by Dexamethasone

1.107 The following tests may be useful in clarifying a diagnosis of premature labour:
    A speculum examination
    B urinary culture
    C plasma progesterone
    D pregnancy test
    E cardiotocography

1.108 The following are associated with preterm labour:
    A bleeding in early pregnancy
    B anencephaly
    C malaria
    D raised serum alpha feto protein
    E Potter's syndrome

(*Answers overleaf*)

1.105 A **False**   Transverse lie in labour should be treated by
B **True**   Caesarean section even if the fetus is dead. If the
C **True**   operator is skilled in such procedures a Blond Heidler
D **True**   saw may be used, but an internal version in these
E **True**   circumstances is very likely to produce a ruptured
uterus. Transverse lie may be due to congenital
uterine abnormalities and may be recurrent and
associated with renal tract abnormalities. A
transverse lie in pregnancy often corrects itself as
term approaches.

E D Morris in Ref 4

1.106 A **False**   Preterm delivery occurs in 5–8% of births in Britain
B **False**   and when associated with fetal or maternal disorders
C **False**   has a better outcome. This may be due to more
D **True**   intensive and prolonged medical supervision or
E **False**   chronic stress inducing fetal maturity. Beta mimetic
drugs may have a place in therapy but not in
prophylaxis. Dexamethasone might accelerate lung
maturity but there is a worrying association with
acute pulmonary oedema when used in conjunction
with beta mimetic drugs.

Ref 8

1.107 A **True**   The early diagnosis of premature labour may be
B **True**   difficult. Abdominal pain may be mild and ignored as
C **False**   insignificant or more severe pain of acute
D **False**   pyelonephritis or appendicitis may be mistaken for
E **True**   labour. Ruptured membranes can be confirmed by a
sterile speculum examination.

K Ritchie & G McClure in Ref 3 Vol 2

1.108 A **True**   Preterm labour is more likely to occur when the
B **True**   pregnancy has been complicated by bleeding.
C **True**   Although anencephaly is associated with
D **True**   postmaturity it is also associated with prematurity as
E **True**   is Potter's syndrome (renal agenesis). Any cause of a
pyrexia may precipitate preterm labour and malaria
is one of the most important world wide. A raised
serum alpha feto protein is found more often than
expected even allowing for the presence of previous
pregnancy complications.

Ref 8

1.109 The following drugs are effective in the treatment of premature labour when compared to a placebo:
A magnesium sulphate
B aminophylline
C dexamethasone
D prostaglandin analogues
E ethanol

1.110 The following drugs are beta sympathomimetic compounds:
A Isoxsuprine
B Indomethacin
C Alcohol
D Terbutaline
E Propanolol

1.111 The following are contra-indications to the use of beta mimetic agents:
A pregnancy at 35 weeks' gestation
B premature membrane rupture
C pre-eclampsia
D ante-partum haemorrhage
E insulin-dependent diabetes

1.112 Beta mimetic drugs are associated with the following side effects:
A increased systolic blood pressure
B increased diastolic blood pressure
C decreased blood sugar
D peripheral vasodilatation
E pyrexia

1.113 The following drugs are first line treatment for these infestations in pregnancy :
A malaria — chloroquine
B toxoplasmosis — pyrimethamine
C schistosoma mansoni — mebendazole
D ankylostoma duodenale — piperazine
E amoebiasis — metronidazole

(*Answers overleaf*)

1.109 A **True**   Ethanol is used with some effect but requires an
     B **False**   unpleasantly high blood level of about 100 mg%.
     C **False**   Aminophylline is not effective. Dexamethasone is
     D **False**   used to induce fetal lung maturity but not to stop
     E **True**   labour. Prostaglandin analogues would stimulate
              labour.

A B M Anderson in Ref 3 Vol 1

1.110 A **True**   Beta sympathomimetic drugs include Isoxuprine,
     B **False**   Ritodrine and Terbutaline. Indomethacin is a
     C **False**   prostaglandin synthetase inhibitor which reduces
     D **True**   uterine contractility. Ethanol also reduces uterine
     E **False**   contractility by a central action. Propanolol is a beta
              adrenergic blocker rather than a beta adrenergic
              agonist.

A B M Anderson in Ref 3 Vol 1

1.111 A **True**   Accepting a reasonable degree of neonatal paediatric
     B **True**   expertise the fetus in all of the above situations is
     C **True**   likely to be at greater risk in utero than in the
     D **True**   neonatal intensive care unit. Current views are that
     E **True**   these drugs should be reserved for use in
              'unexplained' pre term labour in patients who appear
              completely healthy and have a normal healthy fetus
              in utero of less than 34 weeks gestation or weighing
              less then 1500 g. They should have intact membranes
              and a cervix dilated no more than 3 cm.

A B M Anderson in Ref 3 Vol 1

1.112 A **True**   Beta mimetic drugs have important side effects
     B **False**   especially on the cardiovascular system. Pulse rate,
     C **False**   blood pressure, stroke volume and cardiac output all
     D **True**   rise with the consequent strain on cardiac function.
     E **False**   Matermal heart disease must be excluded. Blood
              sugar may increase but only in diabetic patients.

Ref 8

1.113 A **True**   Piperazine should be used for ascaris lumbricoides
     B **True**   (round worm) or enterobius vermicularis (thread
     C **False**   worm), but ankylostoma (hook worm) needs
     D **False**   bephenium or mebendazole particularly if there is a
     E **True**   mixed infestation with whip worm. No anti-malarial
              drug is entirely safe in pregnancy, but chloroquine is
              the best, although quinine might be used in resistant
              cases or for cerebral malaria. All the drugs used for
              schistosomiasis are extremely toxic and treatment
              should wait until after pregnancy.

R Trussell & L Beeley in Ref 5

1.114 Amniotic fluid infection syndrome
- **A** occurs with intact membranes
- **B** is most common in the third trimester of pregnancy
- **C** occurs in poorly nourished pregnant patients
- **D** is related to magnesium deficiency
- **E** occurs because normal amniotic fluid supports bacterial growth

1.115 Eclampsia
- **A** rarely occurs in multiparous patients
- **B** is more common antepartum than postpartum in the United Kingdom
- **C** causes reversible neurological deficit
- **D** should be managed in a darkened room
- **E** causes hyperreflexia

1.116 A 15-year-old primigravida develops blood pressure of 190/110 and proteinuria at 36 weeks gestation. Which of the following drugs would be of value:
- **A** intramuscular Hydralazine
- **B** Salbutamol
- **C** Labetalol
- **D** intravenous infusion of 5% Chlormethiazole (Heminevrin)
- **E** Dexamethasone

1.117 Congenital heart disease complicating pregnancy
- **A** is increasing in incidence
- **B** if due to Eisenmenger's disease entails a high rate of fetal loss
- **C** if due to coarctation of the aorta is an indication for termination of pregnancy
- **D** causes more maternal deaths than acquired heart disease
- **E** is an indication for antibiotic prophylaxis during the antenatal period

(*Answers overleaf*)

1.114 A **True**   Amniotic fluid infection syndrome occurs with intact
     B **False**   membranes in the mid trimester in socially deprived
     C **True**   patients. It is particularly common in
     D **False**   under-privileged black patients in whom an apparent
     E **False**   deficiency of zinc and a polypeptide interfere with the
                   normal bacteriocidal properties of amniotic fluid,
                   most in evidence in the last trimester.

R Schwartz in Ref 3 Vol 2

1.115 A **False**   Although pre eclampsia is mainly a disease of
     B **False**   primigravidae both it and eclampsia occur in
     C **True**   multiparous patients who are likely to have
     D **False**   underlying hypertension. Because of improved
     E **True**   antenatal care eclampsia is now more common post
                   partum than ante partum in the United Kingdom. In
                   Africa the reverse is true. Uncomplicated eclampsia
                   causes irritability of the nervous system and
                   hyperreflexia which are reversible. The possibility of
                   a cerebrovascular accident causing permanent deficit
                   should be considered in serious cases. Eclampsia
                   requires intensive care which cannot be performed in
                   a darkened room. Adequate sedation prevents fits
                   and external stimuli become irrelevant.

Ref 11

1.116 A **False**   Labetalol, 0.8% infusion of Chlormethiazole and
     B **False**   *intravenous* Hydralazine are of value in pre
     C **True**   eclampsia. Intra muscular Hydralazine may produce
     D **False**   an uncontrolled response and is dangerous. There is
     E **False**   no sense in giving Salbutamol or Dexamethasone to
                   a patient at 36 weeks gestation who needs to be
                   delivered and these drugs are also contra indicated
                   with hypertension.

S M Wood in Ref 3 Vol 2

1.117 A **True**   Because an increasing number of these patients have
     B **True**   had surgical correction of their defects in childhood
     C **False**   more are alive and fit to fulfil their reproductive
     D **False**   potential. Eisenmenger's syndrome is one of the
     E **False**   more important causes of fetal and maternal loss.
                   Coarctation of the aorta is relatively benign. Acquired
                   heart disease still causes more maternal deaths than
                   congenital heart disease, although the proportions
                   have been changing.

P Szelely & L Snaith in Ref 5 and Ref 1

1.118 At delivery of twins
A the leading pole is cephalic in 50% of cases
B internal podalic version should be used if the second twin is a breech
C a syntocinon drip should be used in the second stage
D a 2-hour delay between delivery of the twins is acceptable
E the placenta usually separates by the Schultz method

1.119 Induction of labour
A should be performed in borderline cephalo-pelvic disproportion
B should occur in 5%–15% of patients
C needs a higher dose of Syntocinon than augmentation of labour
D can be safely performed for social reasons if the pregnancy is at 41 weeks' gestation and the fetal head 0/5th palpable
E should be monitored by an intra-uterine catheter

1.120 Umbilical cord prolapse is associated with
A multiparity
B footling breech presentation
C post-maturity
D anencephaly
E cephalo-pelvic disproportion

1.121 The management of a patient with umbilical cord prolapse includes
A placing a cord which has emerged from the vulva into the vagina
B placing the patient in an exaggerated Sim's position
C delivery by forceps if fully dilated
D re-positioning of the cord within the uterus
E blood being taken for clotting studies

1.122 The following 18th Century obstetricians wrote classic textbooks of midwifery:
A Mauriceau
B Smellie
C Veit
D Chamberlen
E Denman

(*Answers overleaf*)

1.118 A **False** The leading pole is cephalic in 60-70% of cases at
     B **False** delivery. It is good policy to electively start a
     C **True** syntocinon drip in the second stage as this is
     D **False** commonly required to overcome uterine inertia
     E **True** between delivery of the babies. This period should
not exceed one hour. Perhaps the only indication for
internal podalic version is for transverse or oblique
lie of the second twin with intact or after very
recently ruptured membranes.

Ref 9

1.119 A **False** Induction of labour has in recent years been a much
     B **True** abused technique. It should never be used for
     C **True** cephalo-pelvic disproportion nor for social reasons.
     D **False** There is no indication for induction at 41 weeks if
     E **False** other parameters are normal. The state of the cervix
as well as the validity of the indication is the true
arbiter of 'inducibility' of the patient.

C Hendricks in Ref 3 Vol 3

1.120 A **True** Conditions in which the lower pole of the uterus is
     B **True** not filled by the fetal head or the frank breech
     C **False** predispose to umbilical cord prolapse. Conditions
     D **True** which cause an abnormally large amount of amniotic
     E **True** fluid, such as anencephaly and twin pregnancy, are
also associated with this condition.

Ref 6

1.121 A **True** Steps should be taken to relieve pressure on the cord
     B **True** and to keep it at physiological temperature. If the
     C **True** fetus is alive and the cervix incompletely dilated, then
     D **False** Caesarean section produces the best results, but if
     E **False** the cervix is fully dilated then forceps are
appropriate. Repositioning the cord within the uterus
does not produce good results and clotting studies
are irrelevant.

Ref 6

1.122 A **True** Francois Mauriceau was the author of the most
     B **True** important textbook of its time which ran into eight
     C **False** editions from 1668 till 1752. Many editions were
     D **False** translated by Hugh Chamberlen who strongly
     E **True** criticized the use of the hook and mentioned the
'secret' which he was not prepared to divulge.
William Smellie was a most prolific writer from 1754
until Thomas Denman's book became the most
influential at the turn of the century.

1.123 The following historical comments about instruments are correct:
A the Chamberlen's forceps were described in the late 17th Century
B the vectis was a three-bladed forcep
C the fillet was a single band that was placed around the head of the fetus
D the English lock was introduced by William Smellie
E an early vacuum extractor was described by J Y Simpson

1.124 Which of the following statements about instrumental delivery are true:
A the eighteenth century Chamberlen forceps were closer in design to Kjellands than Neville Barnes forceps
B axis traction may be required for mid cavity forceps
C Kjellands forceps are ideal for the deep transverse arrest in the African patient
D forceps are safer than the vacuum extractor in the presence of excessive caput and moulding
E preliminary assessment of 'station' is more important than abdominal assessment of head level

1.125 Kjelland's forceps
A may be used if the head is two-fifths above the brim
B have no cephalic curve
C have studs on the shank which point towards the sinciput
D have a sliding lock in order to correct asynclitism
E can be used with axis traction

1.126 Shoulder dystocia
A may result in an Erb's palsy, a lesion of C7/8
B is most safely treated by manipulation and internal rotation of the posterior shoulder
C is often preceded by abnormal first stage labour pattern
D is more common with an anencephalic fetus
E is more common in black patients than white patients

(*Answers overleaf*)

1.123 A **False**   Although Peter Chamberlen invented the forceps ·
       B **False**   shortly before 1600, the secret was not made public
       C **True**   until Chapman described them in 1733. The vectis
       D **True**   was single-bladed instrument which was surprisingly
       E **True**   a popular for almost half a century. The fillet as
                     described, was used for obstructed labours. The
                     English lock was introduced by the Scot William
                     Smellie and Simpson in 1849 described a suction
                     traction apparatus.

1.124 A **True**   The Chamberlen forceps, like a pair of metal spoons
       B **False**   without a lock or pelvic curve, were close to Kjellands
       C **False**   forceps. Axis traction or any difficult instrumentation
       D **False**   has no place in modern obstetrics. A vacuum
       E **False**   extractor is safer than forceps in the presence of
                     excessive caput and moulding in the African patient.
                     Abdominal assessment of head level is much more
                     precise and important prognostically than pelvic
                     assessment.

1.125 A **False**   Kjelland's forceps must never be used if the head is
       B **False**   more than one-fifth above brim or with excessive
       C **False**   moulding. Application of blades and rotation should
       D **True**   be uncomplicated and axis traction cannot be used.
       E **False**   The studs point to the occiput and the forceps are
                     useful because of the correction of lateral flexion
                     (asynclitism) and the correction of occipito-posterior
                     and transverse positions.

Ref 6

1.126 A **False**   Shoulder dystocia, a much under-rated obstetric
       B **True**   emergency, may result in an Erb's palsy due to
       C **True**   trauma to the upper roots of the brachial plexus,
       D **True**   C5 & 6. It occurs with a large fetus, which also causes
       E **True**   abnormal progress in the first stage of labour and
                     also with anencephaly. It is best treated by
                     manipulation and rotation of the posterior shoulder
                     and not by the usual custom of pulling laterally on
                     the neck and nerve roots.

Ref 6

1.127 The following statements about epidural block are true:
A it produces perineal hyperaesthesia post partum
B it is indicated in pre eclampsia
C it is safer to continue a successful labour block for Caesarean section than to induce general anaesthesia
D it encourages retained placenta
E it is contra-indicated with abruptio placentae

1.128 A low spinal block
A involves the injection of an anaesthetic agent into the space between the dura membrane and the arachnoid membrane
B acts more slowly than an epidural block
C causes a saddle block
D is complicated by respiratory paralysis
E uses Marcaine

1.129 A classical Caesarean section
A is justified for a prolapsed cord
B is performed through a mid line subumbilical skin incision
C has a high incidence of post-operative pyrexia
D is justified for a repeat Caesarean section
E has a 10% risk of scar rupture in future pregnancies

1.130 Amniotic fluid embolism
A is usually fatal
B characteristically presents before delivery
C occurs more commonly in multiparous patients
D is diagnosed by specific staining techniques
E has been treated with heparin

(Answers overleaf)

1.127 A **True**   Epidural block is a safe means of pain relief for
     B **False**   Caesarean section and it is surprising that
     C **True**   obstetricians usually choose to use a general
     D **False**   anaesthetic even in the presence of a good working
     E **True**   regional block. It is certainly contra-indicated in
accidental haemorrhage and in spite of earlier views
almost certainly contra-indicated in pre-eclampsia,
especially when hypotensive agents are used, as the
effect on the blood pressure may be profound and
unpredictable. The pain of perineal tears is believed
to be more severe after regional block.

J Selwyn-Crawford in Ref 3 Vol 2

1.128 A **False**   Spinal analgesia involves injection of 1% heavy
     B **False**   Nupercaine into the spinal fluid between the
     C **True**   arachnoid and the pia membranes. It acts more
     D **True**   quickly than epidural analgesia but control of its
     E **False**   spread by positional manipulation may be difficult
and if it extends upwards respiratory paralysis,
hypotension and collapse may occur. The area of
anaesthesia produced is known as a saddle block.

J Selwyn-Crawford in Ref 3 Vol 2

1.129 A **False**   A classical Caesarean section is a poor operation with
     B **False**   a higher risk of haematoma, adhesions and infection.
     C **True**   A problem may be caused by African patients visiting
     D **True**   this country and one should beware that a previous
     E **False**   Caesarean section was a classical. Rupture in
approximately 5% of cases often occurs in pregnancy
before labour starts. There are few indications for this
operation, but they include post mortem Caesarean
section, carcinoma of the cervix and occasionally a
transverse lie or a multiple repeat Caesarean section
with dense lower segment adhesions. Hopefully it is
followed by tubal ligation.

J M Beazley in Ref 4

1.130 A **True**   This lethal condition presents before or immediately
     B **False**   after delivery. More common in multiparous patients
     C **True**   having stronger uterine contractions it is ultimately
     D **True**   diagnosed by specific staining of material in the
     E **True**   pulmonary vasculature. There is a clear association
with disseminated intravascular coagulation and
heparin may improve the pulmonary circulation.
Coagulation failure with post partum haemorrhage
may complicate the picture and transfusion with
fresh frozen plasma or specific clotting factors is
indicated.

C R Whitfield in Ref 4

1.131 Rupture of the uterus
   A   is associated with a concealed ante partum haemorrhage
   B   is frequently treated by subtotal hysterectomy
   C   is suggested by a maternal tachycardia in an at-risk case
   D   is a significant danger after myomectomy
   E   is associated with amniotic fluid embolism

1.132 Post partum haemorrhage
   A   is defined as blood loss in excess of 300 ml post partum
   B   is associated with ante partum haemorrhage
   C   is associated with multiple pregnancy
   D   is associated with platelet deficiency
   E   is reduced by the active management of the third stage of
       labour

1.133 Pathological adherence of the placenta is associated with
   A   bicornuate uterus
   B   fetal distress in labour
   C   placenta praevia
   D   previous caesarean section
   E   submucosal myomata

1.134 The following procedures are used to correct uterine inversion:
   A   Helmstein's technique
   B   Spinelli technique
   C   Kustner's technique
   D   hydrostatic manipulation
   E   Haultain technique

(*Answers overleaf*)

1.131 A **True**   Rupture of the uterus is associated with concealed
      B **True**   ante partum haemorrhage and amniotic fluid
      C **True**   embolism. There is little danger of rupture in a uterus
      D **False**   scarred by myomectomy, although other types of
      E **True**   surgery on a pregnant uterus such as hysterotomy do
                    carry a risk.

J M Beazley in Ref 4

1.132 A **False**   The original British definition of post partum
      B **True**   haemorrhage was 20 fluid ounces (570 ml). Most
      C **True**   authorities now accept 500 ml as the correct,
      D **True**   although this is largely irrelevant because any
      E **True**   estimate of post partum loss is inaccurate. Patients
                    with ante partum haemorrhage whether due to
                    accidental haemorrhage or placenta praevia have a
                    tendency to post partum haemorrhage as do those
                    with multiple pregnancy or polyhydramnios. Post
                    partum haemorrhage is occasionally due to a
                    haemostatic defect, or a deficiency of platelets, but is
                    more often due to inadequate uterine contractions
                    and its incidence is reduced by the prophylactic use
                    of ergometrine and delivery of the placenta being
                    expedited.

Ref 6

1.133 A **False**   Pathological adherence of the placenta (termed
      B **False**   placenta accreta, increta or percreta depending on
      C **True**   degree) is associated with previous surgical
      D **True**   procedures involving the uterine cavity such as
      E **True**   Caesarean section, previous manual removal and
                    curettage. Placenta praevia is more likely to be
                    abnormally implanted in the less muscular lower
                    uterine segment. The endometrium covering
                    submucus tumours is said not to decidualise in the
                    normal way.

Ref 6

1.134 A **False**   Hydrostatic manipulation, having ensured there is no
      B **True**   uterine rupture, has been used effectively in this
      C **True**   situation. If manipulation fails then Haultain
      D **True**   technique, using an abdominal approach or Spinelli
      E **True**   or Kustner's technique, using a vaginal approach
                    may be employed to divide the cervix and effect
                    replacement.

Ref 6

1.135 Post partum collapse is a recognised complication of
   A   Addison's disease
   B   phaechromocytoma
   C   hypothyroidism
   D   pre eclampsia
   E   uterine inversion

1.136 Ingestion of drugs during pregnancy causes the following complications in the neonate:
   A   lithium and hypotonus
   B   tricyclic drugs and bradycardia
   C   non-steroidal anti-inflammatory analgesics and prematurity
   D   diazoxide and hyperglycaemia
   E   propranolol and hypoglycaemia

1.137 The following drugs taken by the lactating mother may be harmful to the baby:
   A   heparin
   B   cyclophosphamide
   C   gentamycin
   D   iodides
   E   nicotine

1.138 The fetal alcohol syndrome is associated with
   A   a bone age of less than height age
   B   epicanthic folds
   C   spina bifida
   D   macrosomia
   E   renal abnormalities

(*Answers overleaf*)

1.135 A **True**   Post partum collapse is usually associated with
      B **True**   haemorrhage or sepsis. Patients with Addison's
      C **False**   disease cannot tolerate the stress of delivery with
      D **False**   their inadequate endogenous steroid secretion.
      E **True**   Necrosis of or haemorrhage into a
                     phaeochromocytoma causes collapse because of the
                     loss of adrenergic stimulus.

Ref 6

1.136 A **True**   Lithium toxicity produces hypotonia and cyanosis in
      B **False**   the neonate and the tachycardia, irritability and
      C **False**   tremor following tricyclic anti-depressants are due to
      D **True**   the sympathomimetic and anti-cholinergic effects of
      E **True**   these drugs. Aspirin, indomethacin and naproxen are
                     all inhibitors of prostaglandin synthesis and are
                     associated with a higher incidence of post maturity.
                     Chronic use of diazoxide produces impaired glucose
                     tolerance in the neonate and propranolol produces
                     neonatal bradycardia and hypoglycaemia as a direct
                     effect of beta blockade on the neonate.

L Beeley in Ref 5

1.137 A **False**   Heparin is not present in the breast milk — although
      B **True**   gentamycin is present it probably is not absorbed by
      C **False**   the neonate and ototoxicity has not been reported.
      D **True**   Cytotoxic drugs have produced neutropenia in a
      E **True**   breast-fed child. Iodides including those found in
                     cough mixtures produce hypothyroidism and goitre.
                     The smoking of 20 cigarettes a day may decrease
                     lactation and cause jitteriness in the baby.

L Beeley in Ref 5

1.138 A **False**   The fetal alcohol syndrome, first reported by Jones in
      B **True**   1973, produces small for dates infants with
      C **False**   permanent stunting of growth, a characteristic facies,
      D **False**   microcephaly, mental defect, cardiac and renal
      E **True**   abnormalities. The syndrome follows excessive
                     drinking of any type of alcohol, either as steady
                     drinking or bingeing. It also follows a regular small
                     input, therefore drinking in pregnancy should be
                     discouraged as firmly as smoking.

Ref 16

1.139 A third degree tear
A is more common with a central episiotomy
B should be repaired under general anaesthesia
C should have the anal sphincter repaired before the vagina
D should have prophylactic antibiotics
E may lead to a vesico-vaginal fistulae

1.140 Internal iliac artery ligation
A causes necrosis of pelvic tissue
B arrests blood flow in a severed uterine artery
C is useful in the treatment of post partum haemorrhage
D is performed just below the origin of the ovarian artery
E is useful in the treatment of broad ligament haematoma

1.141 Coagulation defects are associated with
A hydatidiform mole
B fulminating pre-eclampsia
C red degeneration of a fibroid
D acute inversion of the uterus
E amniotic fluid embolism

1.142 Bleeding which occurs on the fifth post-partum day
A requires ergometrine
B may be due to a carneous mole
C requires an evacuation of the uterus
D should be investigated by ultrasound
E is associated with subsequent infertility

(*Answers overleaf*)

1.139 A **True**   Although a central episiotomy is more comfortable
       B **False**   and the patient has less blood loss, third degree tear
       C **True**   is very common. Repair under local anaesthesia with
       D **False**   good retraction and illumination is adequate and the
       E **False**   rectal and anal components of the tear should be
                       repaired first. There is a danger of a recto-vaginal
                       fistula but good technique and haemostasis rather
                       than prophylactic antibiotics will prevent this
                       breakdown.

Ref 6

1.140 A **False**   Internal iliac artery ligation performed after division
       B **False**   of the peritoneum and mobilization of the ureter at
       C **True**   the level of the bifurcation of the common iliac artery
       D **False**   is effective treatment for intractable post partum
       E **True**   haemorrhage or broad ligament haematoma.
                       Adequate collateral circulation exists not to
                       compromise the viability of pelvic tissue and to
                       maintain some flow through the uterine artery
                       although at reduced pressure. The origin of the
                       ovarian artery is from the aorta or renal artery well
                       above the site of intervention.

J M Beazley in Ref 4

1.141 A **False**   There is an association of disseminated intravascular
       B **True**   coagulation with intra uterine death, missed
       C **False**   abortion, ante partum haemorrhage, amniotic fluid
       D **False**   embolism and pre-eclampsia. However, a laboratory
       E **True**   diagnosis of coagulation defect does not mean
                       troublesome bleeding will occur and therapy should
                       be held in reserve.

C R Whitfield in Ref 4

1.142 A **False**   Secondary post-partum haemorrhage is almost
       B **False**   always due to retained placental tissue. It is
       C **True**   associated with secondary infertility because of
       D **False**   associated pelvic infection and should be treated by
       E **True**   surgical evacuation rather than ergometrine. Clinical
                       assessment should be adequate to make the
                       diagnosis and ultrasonic investigation is
                       unnecessary.

Ref 6

1.143 The following are indications for a 7-day course of antibiotics post partum:
A   a temperature of 38.0 °C two days after a Caesarean section.
B   deep venous thrombosis
C   manual removal of placenta
D   rheumatic heart disease
E   prolonged premature membrane rupture before delivery.

1.144 Colostrum
A   is alkaline
B   contains less protein than breast milk
C   contains less carbohydrate than breast milk
D   contains less sodium than breast milk
E   contains antibodies

1.145 The following statements concerning lactation are correct:
A   using alternate breasts for successive feeds enhances lactation
B   'resting the breasts' helped by supplementation with artificial feeds in the first few days enhances lactation
C   prolactin secretion increases during suckling
D   the suckling reflex stimulates milk secretion
E   prostaglandins are involved in milk ejection

1.146 The following statements concerning breast fed infants compared with bottle fed infants are correct:
A   obesity is more common
B   allergic disorders are more common
C   childhood cancer is less common
D   sudden infant death syndrome (cot death) is less common
E   gastro intestinal infection is less common

1.147 The following factors discourage 'bonding':
A   low socio-economic group
B   ultrasonic examination
C   episiotomy
D   forceps delivery
E   neonatal intensive care

(Answers overleaf)

1.143
A **False**
B **False**
C **True**
D **False**
E **True**

Antibiotics are overprescribed and the indication for their use should be clear. A temperature of 38 °C is common after any major operation, and is likely to be due to re-absorption of blood or necrotic tissue. An established infection or a situation where intra-uterine infection is likely, such as manual removal of the placenta or prolonged membrane rupture, with consequent risk to fertility necessitates their use. Prophylactic antibiotics to cover delivery in a cardiac patient should be discontinued after 48 hours.

1.144
A **True**
B **False**
C **True**
D **False**
E **True**

Colostrum is an alkaline yellow secretion. It has nutritive value containing more protein and less carbohydrate than breast milk. It transfers antibodies to the fetus and plays a part in the establishment of neonatal immune status. It also has a natural laxative action.

Ref 12

1.145
A **False**
B **False**
C **True**
D **False**
E **False**

After priming during pregnancy with oestrogen and progesterone it is prolactin which is the essential hormone in maintaining lactation being augmented by suckling. Maximal suckling stimulation and emptying of the milk is desirable to maintain milk production. Suckling does not directly stimulate the acini but induces oxytocin release which stimulates the myoepithelial cells to eject the milk.

Ref 12

1.146
A **False**
B **False**
C **False**
D **True**
E **True**

Amongst the many advantages of breast feeding convenience, cheapness and reduction of gastro intestinal infection are the most important. There is evidence of a decreased incidence of allergic disorders such as asthma and eczema in breast fed babies, fewer cot deaths and less obesity.

Ref 12

1.147
A **True**
B **False**
C **True**
D **True**
E **True**

The most potent factor against bonding is the unwillingness of a mother to be pregnant. This may be due to unemployment, not being married or being in the low income group. Ultrasonic examination almost certainly encourages bonding and the principal obstetric adverse factors are those which decrease the involvement of the mother in the perinatal period.

A Reading in Ref 3 Vol 3

1.148 The following signs would contribute to the lowering of the Apgar score:
A fetal pulse of 120 per minute
B pallor
C respiration 30 per minute
D absence of Moro reflex
E irregular respiration

1.149 In the management of stillbirth
A spontaneous labour should be awaited
B the mother should be discouraged from touching the baby
C lactation should be suppressed with bromocriptine
D glucose tolerance test should be performed before discharge from hospital
E attempts to conceive as soon as possible should be discouraged

1.150 The following vessels contain oxygenated blood in the fetus:
A umbilical artery
B ductus venosus
C the inferior vena cava as it enters the right atrium
D carotid artery
E umbilical vein

1.151 In the fetal circulation there is:
A right to left shunting at atrial level
B left to right shunting at ductal level
C greater oxygen saturation in the left hepatic lobe of blood supply than the right
D oxygen saturation of blood entering the fetal lung is low
E ductal flow which can be abolished by prostaglandin synthetase inhibitors

(*Answers overleaf*)

1.148 A **False**   Fetal heart beat of 120 and respiration of 30 per
     B **True**   minute each scored 2. Pallor scored zero. Irregular
     C **False**   respirations score 1 and reflex activity is tested by
     D **False**   grimace on stimulation and not the Moro reflex.
     E **True**

Ref 6

1.149 A **False**   It is an unreasonable psychological stress for a
     B **False**   patient with an intra uterine death to await
     C **True**   spontaneous delivery. Modern induction methods
     D **False**   should ensure delivery whatever the length of
     E **True**   gestation or the state of the cervix. Seeing and
touching the baby will facilitate mourning. It is kind
to suppress lactation with the most efficient means
available and discharge patients from hospital,
especially the obstetric unit, without delay. A
reasonable interval before subsequent pregnancy
should be encouraged because psychological
problems are less likely if the subsequent pregnancy
is not used as a replacement for the unsuccessful
one.

1.150 A **False**   The umbilical vein carries oxygenated blood from the
     B **True**   placenta to the fetus. This blood then flows through
     C **True**   the liver, or bypasses it through the ductus venosus,
     D **True**   and then enters the inferior vena cava. Blood
     E **True**   entering the heart from the inferior vena cava is
shunted through the foramen ovale into the left
atrium. From the left ventricle it is ejected into the
ascending aorta to provide a good supply of
oxygenated blood to the brain, coronary arteries and
upper extremities. Ultimately deoxygenated blood
returns to the placenta through the umbilical artery.

Ref 15

1.151 A **True**   Two-thirds of inferior vena caval flow is directed to
     B **False**   the left but two-thirds of right heart output goes to
     C **True**   the aorta. The left lobe of the liver receives
     D **True**   oxygenated blood from the umbilical vein and the
     E **True**   right lobe receives venous blood from the portal vein.
This may explain the occasional finding of
degenerative changes on the right side.
Indomethacin may close the ductus arteriosus but
this is not always effective.

Ref 16

1.152 Down's syndrome
- A is Trisomy 23
- B may be a translocation abnormality carrying a 1 in 10 risk for female carriers
- C occurs more frequently in a patient with a history of previously affected offspring than in patients over 40 years old
- D occurs in 1% of pregnancies with a maternal age of 40 years
- E is associated with paternal age

1.153 Patau's syndrome
- A is Trisomy D
- B occurs once in 5000 births
- C is characterized by cleft palate and polydactyly
- D have typical cri du chat characteristics
- E has been diagnosed by fetoscopy

1.154 Edwards syndrome
- A is Trisomy 18
- B is associated with abnormal feet
- C is not age related
- D has a mortality of 50% by two months of age
- E have microcephaly

1.155 Amniocentesis
- A precipitates abortion
- B is easily performed at twelve weeks gestation
- C is used in the prenatal diagnosis of spina bifida
- D is associated with neonatal postural limb defects
- E should be followed by anti-D immunoglobulin injection in Rhesus negative mothers

(*Answers overleaf*)

1.152 A **False**   Down's syndrome, which is Trisomy 21 in 90% of
      B **True**   cases, may also be a translocation between
      C **False**   chromosomes 15 and 21. Maternal age is the most
      D **True**   important factor in trisomic fetuses with a risk of 1%
      E **True**   at age 40 years and 3% at age 45 years. In younger
women translocation occurs more frequently but
nevertheless in the individual case a trisomic
abnormality is more probable. There is also an
association with paternal age over 55 years, previous
Down's offspring and a parent having a translocation
or mosaic genotype.

Ref 16

1.153 A **True**   Patau's syndrome is trisomy 13 or D trisomy and is
      B **False**   the third major autosomal abnormality observed in
      C **True**   the neonatal period with an incidence of 1:20 000.
      D **False**   The abnormalities are variable but include severe
      E **False**   mental retardation, congenital heart disease,
abnormal ears, polydactyly, cleft palate and
holoprosencephaly varying in severity sometimes as
extreme as cyclopia. The cri du chat syndrome is
typically a deletion of the short arm of chromosome 5
and is not related to Patau's syndrome. Patau's
syndrome has not been diagnosed by fetoscopy.

Ref 16

1.154 A **True**   Trisomy 18 or E trisomy is the second most common
      B **True**   autosomal abnormality occurring more often in
      C **False**   females (4 to 1). Rocker bottom feet, cleft lip and
      D **True**   palate and flexion deformities of the fingers are
      E **False**   recognised features. 50% die by two months and 90%
die by one year. Although uniformly severely
mentally retarded microcephaly is not a feature. Like
all trisomies they are related to maternal age.

M A Stenchever in Ref 12

1.155 A **True**   Amniocentesis has been shown to carry an increased
      B **False**   risk of abortion, postural limb defects and
      C **True**   sensitization of rhesus negative mothers. It is not
      D **True**   possible or easy until fourteen to sixteen weeks
      E **True**   gestation as there is not enough liquor and the
fundus is not easily palpable per abdomen. Amniotic
fluid alphafetoprotein is measured in patients at risk
for spina bifida. Counselling is important as one must
be sure that the probability of a detectable affected
pregnancy is significantly greater than the probability
of aborting a normal pregnancy.

J S Scott in Ref 4

1.156 Intrauterine fetal transfusion
- **A** uses packed O Rh Negative blood
- **B** should not be performed if premature labour threatened
- **C** may be performed by fetoscopy
- **D** is not performed before 22 weeks
- **E** is monitored by maternal OD 450

1.157 Rhesus iso-immunization
- **A** only occurs when the father is homozygous for Rhesus factor
- **B** only occurs with Rhesus negative mothers
- **C** only occurs with Rhesus positive offspring
- **D** requires the feto-maternal transfusion of at least 5 mls of blood
- **E** is less likely to occur when there is ABO incompatibility between mother and child

1.158 The following are transient and benign findings on examination of the neonate:
- **A** hepatomegaly
- **B** cataracts
- **C** milia
- **D** subconjunctival haemorrhages
- **E** mongolian spots

1.159 Mechanisms involved in the maintenance of body temperature in a mature neonate include:
- **A** sweating
- **B** changes in skin blood flow
- **C** shivering
- **D** increase in physical activity
- **E** metabolism of brown fat

(*Answers overleaf*)

1.156 A **True**   Fetal transfusion uses O Rh Negative blood packed to
      B **False** haemoglobin 24 g/dl and compatible with the
      C **True**   mother, although with fetoscopy the fetal blood
      D **True**   group may be found and the appropriate ABO
      E **False** grouped blood given on future occasions. It is in the
                   fetal interest to proceed with scheduled transfusion
                   despite vaginal bleeding, ruptured membranes or
                   threatened premature labour. Transfusion is
                   performed between 22 and 35 weeks and direct
                   transfusion into an umbilical vessel via the fetoscope
                   has been described.

C R Whitfield in Ref 3 Vol 2

1.157 A **False** Only one paternal gene is required and therefore a
      B **True**   heterozygous father can supply the D gene to the
      C **True**   fetus. A trans-placental bleed of much less than 5 ml
      D **False** of blood may immunize the fetus particularly if
      E **True**   mother and child are of the same ABO blood group.

C R Whitfield in Ref 3 Vol 2

1.158 A **True**   Hepatomegaly, milia (white spots on the nose) and
      B **False** subconjunctival haemorrhages are common benign
      C **True**   findings in the neonate. Congenital cataracts are
      D **True**   always abnormal and a search for a cause should
      E **True**   always be made. Mongolian spots are slate blue, well
                   demarcated areas of pigmentation usually on the
                   back. They are seen in non-white and mixed race
                   infants and disappear within a year.

Ref 17

1.159 A **False** Neonates do not sweat effectively or shiver, but
      B **True**   metabolise brown fat which accounts for about 5% of
      C **False** the neonatal body weight to produce heat. The
      D **True**   neonate is at great risk from temperature changes
      E **True**   and must be dried immediately, clothed and placed
                   in a warm environment. Premature neonates are
                   especially prone to hypothermia. Overhead radiant
                   heaters, foil wrapping and prewarmed incubators are
                   essential in the labour ward.

Ref 15

1.160 Neonatal jaundice
A occurring within the first twenty-four hours of life is usually physiological
B does not require treatment unless the concentration of unconjugated bilirubin is more than 20 mg% (340 µmol/l)
C is treated by phototherapy using light of wavelength 400 to 500 nanometers
D is treated by exchange transfusion
E causes kernicterus by the deposition of free conjugated bilirubin in the brain

1.161 Neonatal jaundice is associated with:
A galactosaemia
B sickle cell disease (Hb SS)
C breast feeding
D hypothyroidism
E achondroplasia

1.162 Idiopathic respiratory distress syndrome in the neonate
A is associated with low birth weight
B usually begins four days after birth
C is associated with maternal diabetes mellitus
D may be prevented by administration of corticosteroids to a patient with threatened premature labour between twenty-eight and thirty-four weeks' gestation
E is commoner in neonates born by Caesarean section

1.163 Recognized complications in light for date babies include:
A polycythaemia
B increased gastro-intestinal infection
C meconium aspiration
D poor feeding
E hypogylcaemia

(*Answers overleaf*)

1.160 A **False** Physiological jaundice appears after the first
      B **False** twenty-four hours of life, reaching a peak about the
      C **True**   fourth day and disappearing within seven days. The
      D **True**   peak level of physiological jaundice is generally
      E **False** below 12 mg% and treatment is indicated at a level of
                   15 mg% in a premature baby and 20 mg% in a term
                   baby, and treatment by phototherapy, which is aimed
                   at preventing exchange transfusion starts at
                   12–15 mg% in a term baby. The danger of bilirubin is
                   the deposition of free unconjugated bilirubin
                   (kernicterus) in the basal ganglia causing cerebral
                   palsy with abnormal movements, deafness and
                   mental retardation.

Ref 15

1.161 A **True**   The association of jaundice and cataracts in a
      B **False** neonate suggests a diagnosis of galactosaemia
      C **True**   which may be detected by a simple heel prick blood
      D **True**   test. Sickle cell disease which may include jaundice
      E **False** as a feature in the older child does not cause
                   neonatal problems. The cause of breast milk
                   jaundice is obscure but a steroid present in the milk
                   may be responsible. Persistent jaundice after seven
                   days is an indication for thyroid studies; other signs
                   of hypothyroidism such as hypotonia and umbilical
                   hernia may be absent and early treatment is
                   essential.

Ref 18

1.162 A **True**   Idiopathic respiratory distress syndrome, hyaline
      B **False** membrane disease, is commoner in preterm
      C **True**   neonates, those of diabetic mothers at all gestations
      D **True**   and those born by Caesarean section. Liggins and
      E **True**   Howie in New Zealand have produced evidence that
                   it may be prevented by the administration of
                   corticosteroids. It always begins soon after birth and
                   is recognized by tachypnoea, grunting and intercostal
                   recession.

Ref 18

1.163 A **True**   Polycythaemia, gasping and hence meconium
      B **False** aspiration and also hypoglycaemia following
      C **True**   mobilization of the liver glycogen are all the result of
      D **False** prolonged hypoxia and intra uterine malnutrition.
      E **True**   The immune mechanisms are normal and light for
                   dates infants typically feed well.

J K Ritchie & G McClure in Ref 3 Vol 1

1.164 The following tests require knowledge of the patient's last menstrual period
    A serum alpha feto protein
    B shake test
    C urinary oestriols
    D oxytocin stress test
    E rubella haemoglutination inhibition test

1.165 The congenital Rubella syndrome
    A may be prevented by vaccination in early pregnancy
    B causes intra-uterine growth retardation
    C causes cataracts
    D causes deafness only if acquired before 16 weeks of gestation
    E can be diagnosed by a rise in maternal IgA

1.166 Intra uterine growth retardation is characteristically associated with
    A maternal diabetes mellitus
    B cervical incompetence
    C pre-eclampsia
    D intra uterine infection
    E multiple pregnancy

1.167 Meconium aspiration syndrome in the neonate
    A causes a chemical pneumonitis
    B causes changes on chest X ray
    C is associated with pneumomediastinum
    D is treated by lung lavage using 5% dextrose
    E is treated by positive pressure ventilation as first choice

(*Answers overleaf*)

1.164 A **True**   Only serum alphafetoprotein and urinary oestriol
      B **False**   require the date of the last menstrual period for
      C **True**   interpretation.
      D **False**
      E **False**

1.165 A **False**   Infection of a mother with rubella in early pregnancy
      B **True**   causes symmetrical intra-uterine growth retardation,
      C **True**   congenital heart disease, cataracts, microcephaly and
      D **False**   thrombocytopaenia if the disease is acquired before
      E **False**   16 weeks. Deafness, however, may be detected in
                      fetuses whose mothers have acquired rubella as late
                      as 22 weeks. The disease is detected in mothers by a
                      rise in Rubella-specific IgM and is largely preventable
                      by vaccination at least 3 months before pregnancy.

A Harvey & I Kovar in Ref 3 Vol 1

1.166 A **True**   Babies of diabetic mothers may be large, particularly
      B **False**   if the diabetes has not been well controlled although
      C **True**   growth retardation occurs if there is nephropathy.
      D **True**   Cervical incompetence leading to premature delivery
      E **True**   will result in a small neonate appropriate for
                      gestational age. Pre-eclampsia causes growth
                      retardation due to poor placental function. Intra
                      uterine infection causes growth retardation by
                      placental damage and by infection of the fetus itself
                      causing poor growth potential. Fetuses in multiple
                      pregnancy may be small because of increased
                      demand on the placenta.

H R Gamsu in Ref 7

1.167 A **True**   Meconium aspiration syndrome is associated with
      B **True**   growth retardation and asphyxia usually in mature
      C **True**   babies. Opacities may be seen on radiological
      D **False**   examination of the chest. Pneumothorax and
      E **False**   pneumomediastinum occur. It may be prevented by
                      careful management of the at risk fetus by
                      nasopharyngeal suction before delivery of the body
                      and lung lavage should be performed with saline (5%
                      Dextrose is toxic). Positive pressure ventilation
                      should only be used as a last resort and high
                      concentrations of humidified oxygen in a head box
                      are preferable.

Ref 15

1.168 Pneumothorax in a neonate occurs in association with
  A meconium aspiration syndrome
  B pneumonia
  C idiopathic respiratory distress syndrome
  D transient tachypnoea of the newborn
  E positive pressure ventilation during resuscitation

1.169 Microcephaly
  A is produced by cytomegalo virus infection
  B results from alcohol abuse
  C results from excessive maternal smoking
  D is incompatible with life after infancy
  E is associated with fetal growth retardation

1.170 Downs syndrome is characteristically associated with:
  A patent ductus arteriosus
  B pyloric stenosis
  C Brushfield's spots
  D congenital cataracts
  E maternal drug abuse

1.171 The following karyotypes are appropriate:
  A 45, X/46, XX — Turner mosaic
  B 47, XXt13 — Patau's syndrome
  C 46, XY 5p — Cri-du-chat syndrome
  D 47, XYY — Klinefelter's syndrome
  E 45, XXt (14q 21q) — Balanced translocation carrier for Down's syndrome

(*Answers overleaf*)

1.168 A **True**   If deterioration occurs in respiratory function in a
      B **True**   case of meconium aspiration, idiopathic respiratory
      C **True**   distress syndrome, or if resuscitation was necessary,
      D **False**   pneumothorax must be excluded by radiological
      E **True**   examination. Pneumonia causes hyperventilation
                     and plugging of the bronchi, both of which may
                     produce rupture of peripheral alveoli.

Ref 15

1.169 A **True**   Microcephaly may result from infection with the
      B **True**   TORCH group of viruses (Toxoplasmosis, Rubella,
      C **False**   Cytomegalo virus, Herpes virus), syphilis, fetal
      D **False**   alcohol syndrome, congenital abnormalities and
      E **True**   some cytotoxic drugs. These factors also produce
                     fetal growth retardation. Patients with microcephaly
                     often survive with variable mental and physical
                     handicaps. The diagnosis may be made at 20 weeks
                     by serial ultrasound examinations.

I Kovar & D Harvey in Ref 3

1.170 A **True**   Congenital heart disease especially ventricular septal
      B **False**   defect is associated with Down's syndrome. Patent
      C **True**   ductus arteriosis is the third most common heart
      D **False**   defect associated with Downs syndrome following
      E **False**   VSD and ASD frequency. Congenital cataracts are not
                     one of the common manifestations. The
                     characteristic intestinal abnormality is duodenal
                     atresia. Brushfield's spots which are pale speckles on
                     the iris occur in 50% of cases.

C Scully in Ref 7

1.171 A **True**   'a' is usually a classical phenotype, 'b' is Trisomy 13,
      B **True**   'c' is partial short arm deletion 'd' is the extra Y
      C **True**   male who may have behavioural problems —
      D **False**   Klinefelters is 47 XXY. 'e' is a balanced translocation
      E **True**   (t) with fusion of a 14q and a 21q and is hence a
                     carrier of Down's syndrome.

Ref 18

1.172 The following statements about sex chromosome trisomies are appropriate:
A   47 XXX are of short stature
B   47 XXX have mental retardation
C   47 XXY are always infertile
D   47 XYY have an increased incidence of congenital heart disease
E   The offspring of 47 XYY are normal

1.173 Intraventricular haemorrhage of the newborn
A   is the most common example of intracranial haemorrhage
B   is associated with respiratory distress syndrome
C   is characteristically associated with birth injury
D   causes apnoeic attacks
E   is preventable by routine correction of coagulation disturbances

1.174 Fetoscopy has been successfully used for the prenatal diagnosis of
A   thalassaemia
B   epidermolysis bullosa
C   Treacher-Collins syndrome
D   Christmas disease (haemophilia B)
E   Duchenne muscular dystrophy

1.175 An abnormal number of digits occurs with
A   Patau's syndrome
B   amniotic bands
C   Down's syndrome
D   Laurence-Moon-Biedl syndrome
E   gentamycin therapy

(*Answers overleaf*)

1.172 A **False**   Patients with the triple X syndrome have no
       B **True**   characteristic physical features. They are of normal
       C **True**   fertility but usually have some degree of mental
       D **False**   retardation. Uniformly the offspring have been
       E **True**   normal — this seems strange as meiosis should
                      produce ova containing one or two X chromosomes.
                      Apart from a reputation for aggressive anti-social
                      behaviour, men with 47 XYY have no other special
                      features.

R P Shearman in Ref 4

1.173 A **True**   Intraventricular haemorrhage is twice as common as
       B **True**   other types of cerebral haemorrhage. It is a common
       C **False**   occurrence in babies dying of respiratory distress
       D **True**   syndrome and causes apnoeic attacks, usually with
       E **False**   flaccidity and cyanosis. Birth injury causes other
                      types of intracranial haemorrhage and
                      intraventricular bleeding is not preventable by
                      correction of coagulation abnormalities, although
                      these are often present.

Ref 6

1.174 A **True**   Fetal blood sampling by fetoscopy has provided the
       B **True**   numerically most important prenatal diagnosis of
       C **True**   blood disorders. Thalassaemia, sickle cell disease and
       D **True**   haemophilia may be diagnozed. The abnormal neck
       E **False**   and head of Treacher-Collins syndrome has been
                      visualized and skin biosy has permitted a diagnosis
                      of epidermolysis bullosa. Duchenne muscular
                      dystrophy remains a problem as creatine
                      phosphokinase levels of fetal blood are variable and
                      muscle biopsy has not been performed.

C H Rodeck in Ref 3

1.175 A **True**   Polydactyly defined as more than five digits per hand
       B **True**   occurs in many syndromes including Patau's
       C **False**   syndrome and Laurence-Moon-Biedl syndrome. It is
       D **True**   also a frequent isolated abnormality. Syndactyly
       E **False**   defined as fusion or webbing of the fingers occurs as
                      an isolated defect. Amniotic bands cause a variety of
                      amputation deformities depending on their site.

Ref 16

1.176 Cephalopelvic disproportion in the absence of gross pelvic abnormality can be diagnosed by
A   ultrasound
B   a maternal stature of less than 158 cm
C   trial of labour
D   x-ray pelvimetry
E   pelvic examination

1.177 The following statements about cervimetric pattern in primigravida are correct:
A   a normal cervimetric curve is associated with a 1–2% Caesarean section rate
B   the prolonged latent phase has a 1–5% Caesarean section rate
C   primary dysfunctional labour occurs in 5–15% of labours
D   primary dysfunctional labour corrected by Syntocinon has a Caesarean section rate of 5–10%
E   augmented secondary arrest may produce uterine rupture

1.178 Erect X-ray lateral pelvimetry
A   is necessary for the diagnosis of cephalo-pelvic disproportion
B   will reveal the bi-spinous diameter
C   should be performed for failure to progress in active labour
D   should be performed if spontaneous labour occurs at 34 weeks gestation with a breech presentation
E   should be performed before induction of labour if there are doubts about the adequacy of the pelvis

1.179 The following statements about breech presentation are correct:
A   labour should be induced at term
B   augmentation of dysfunctional labour by oxytocic drugs should be avoided
C   cerebral haemorrhage is the most common cause of perinatal death
D   external cephalic version should be avoided
E   the fetus weighing 1000–1500 g should be delivered by Caesarean section

(Answers overleaf)

1.176 A **False**   Factors which make one suspect cephalopelvic
     B **False**   disproportion are short stature, small pelvis, high
     C **True**   head at term and a previous difficult delivery, but the
     D **False**   only way to diagnose cephalopelvic disproportion is
     E **False**   by a well-conducted trial of labour with good uterine
                    contractions.

J W W Studd, L D Cardozo, D M F Gibb in Ref 3 Vol 2

1.177 A **True**   Primigravidae with a normal cervimetric pattern has
     B **False**   approximately a 1–5% incidence of Caesarean
     C **False**   section, but prolonged latent phase has a much
     D **True**   higher incidence of between 5–15%. Primary
     E **False**   dysfunctional labour occurs in approximately 30% of
                    labours and if augmented improves with Syntocinon,
                    the Caesarean section rate should be between
                    5–10%. Although the secondary arrest is
                    characteristically a treacherous complication in
                    multigravid patients, a primigravid uterus should not
                    rupture following augmentation.

J W W Studd, L D Cardozo, D M F Gibb in Ref 3 Vol 2

1.178 A **False**   Cephalo-pelvic disproportion is a functional
     B **False**   diagnosis made by a trial of labour with good
     C **False**   contractions and not by X-ray examination. This
     D **False**   investigation has a diminishing place in obstetric
     E **False**   practice but should be used in the assessment of a
                    primigravid breech presentation and in the
                    assessment of a patient with a previous Caesarean
                    section.

J W W Studd, L D Cardozo & D M F Gibb in Ref 3 Vol 2

1.179 A **False**   Fetal malformation is by far the most common cause
     B **True**   of perinatal death. Labour should not be induced
     C **False**   because of the breech presentation and any slowness
     D **False**   in the first stage is an indication for Caesarean
     E **True**   section. Fetal weight gained between 40 weeks and
                    42 weeks is not sufficient to allow a difference in
                    weight to be an indication for induction of labour.
                    External cephalic version has a place if the
                    procedure is easy and there are no contra-indications
                    such as previous uterine scar or a Rhesus negative
                    maternal blood group. Literature concerning
                    Caesarean section and the small breech remains
                    confused, but there is a consensus that the fetus
                    weighing between 1000 and 1500 g is delivered in
                    better condition by Caesarean section.

N Duignan Ref 3

1.180 Forceps can be safely used for delivery
  A   only if the rectum and bladder are empty
  B   if the head is two-fifths above the pelvic brim
  C   if the Mentovertical diameter is presenting
  D   before full dilatation using Duhrssens incisions
  E   if the scalp is showing at the vulva

1.181 The vacuum extractor (Ventouse)
  A   is safely used for traction for up to 20 minutes
  B   is useful when there is caput and moulding
  C   should be placed near to the posterior fontanelle
  D   can be used when the head is two-fifths palpable above the pelvic brim
  E   is most effective when used with an epidural block

1.182 In coagulation failure in obstetrics
  A   fibrin degradation products have an anticoagulant effect
  B   thromboplastin deficiency is common
  C   emptying the uterus is a priority
  D   standard blood transfusion is therapeutic
  E   the platelet count is depressed

(*Answers overleaf*)

1.180 A **False**   It is unusual for the rectum as well as the bladder to
     B **False**   be empty and it is not particularly important. Forceps
     C **False**   are safe if the head is 0/5th or 1/5th palpable
     D **False**   abdominally — not higher — and it is possible in
     E **False**   cephalo-pelvic disproportion for caput to be visible at
the vulva and the head 2/5th palpable above the
brim. Brow presentation has a Mentovertical
diameter of 13 cm and should be delivered
abdominally. Duhrssens incisions are claimed to be
useful in cases of acute fetal distress, a head deeply
engaged and the cervix offering the only obstruction
to delivery. However, the dangers of uterine damage
are too great for it to be used.

Ref H Philpot in Ref 3 Vol 3

1.181 A **False**   The vacuum extractor should be applied as far
     B **True**   posterior as possible and may be used as a trial of
     C **True**   vacuum in theatre if there is caput and moulding with
     D **True**   the head two-fifths palpable above the pelvic brim.
     E **False**   Good maternal effort increases the safety of the
instrument, hence an epidural does not facilitate its
successful use. Traction should be applied during
three contractions only and traction for 20 minutes is
excessive in spite of the apparent approval of 40
minutes in some standard texts. It is usually quite
clear during that time whether the baby will be
delivered safely or not.

H Philpot in Ref 3 Vol 3

1.182 A **True**   The common factor in conditions causing
     B **False**   coagulation failure in obstetrics is thromboplastin
     C **True**   released from the uterine contents, or damaged
     D **False**   tissues. Fibrinolysis generates fibrin degradation
     E **True**   products which themselves inhibit coagulation.
Platelets are consumed by the coagulation process. A
standard blood transfusion is not helpful as it does
not contain clotting factors and fresh blood, fresh
frozen plasma or cryoprecipitates must be used.

C R Whitfield in Ref 4

1.183 The following factors affect birth weight
A   parity
B   acute malnutrition
C   environmental altitude
D   ethnic origin
E   'dieting'

1.184 The following conditions may be diagnosed prenatally using a sample of amniotic fluid:
A   Tay-Sachs disease
B   phenyl ketonuria
C   Duchenne muscular dystrophy
D   cystinosis
E   Neimann-Pick disease

1.185 Fetal ascites is associated with
A   fetal aortic stenosis
B   ABO incompatibility
C   nephrosis
D   cystic adenomatoid lung malformation
E   spontaneous regression

1.186 Gestational age in the neonate is accurately assessed by
A   weight charts for respective sexes
B   period of maternal amenorrhoea
C   Apgar scoring system
D   Dubowitz scoring system
E   head circumference measurement

(*Answers overleaf*)

1.183 A **True**   Many factors have some effect on birth weight.
      B **True**   Parous patients tend to have bigger babies and
      C **True**   babies resulting from multiple conceptions are
      D **True**   smaller. Heavy smokers have smaller babies as do
      E **False**   people living in high altitude. Genetic and ethnic
                    influences are clearly important and Asian patients
                    produce smaller babies. Dieting, unless extreme,
                    does not have any effect on fetal weight but acute
                    starvation in previously well-nourished women as in
                    Holland during the Second World War resulted in
                    growth retarded babies.

J Wilcocks in Ref 14

1.184 A **True**   Studying the metabolic activity of cells cultured from
      B **False**   amniotic fluid has permitted the prenatal diagnosis of
      C **False**   many biochemical errors of metabolism. Tay-Sachs
      D **True**   disease, cystinosis and Niemann-Pick disease may be
      E **True**   diagnosed in this way. However, the enzyme
                    involved in phenyl ketonuria is not present even in
                    the amniotic fluid of normal fetuses and a fetus with
                    Duchenne muscular dystrophy has no specific
                    amniotic marker.

D Harvey in Ref 7

1.185 A **True**   Fetal ascites now diagnosed with increasing
      B **False**   frequency by ultrasonic investigation is associated
      C **True**   with many fetal disorders. However idiopathic cases
      D **True**   occur and spontaneous regression has been
      E **True**   reported. Persisting ascites is one of the features of
                    hydrops fetalis.

Ref 16

1.186 A **False**   The Dubowitz scoring system is one of several
      B **False**   methods available for the assessment of gestational
      C **False**   maturity of the neonate. It involves the assessment of
      D **True**   twelve physical and ten neurological criteria. Head
      E **False**   circumference and weight charts are unreliable
                    because of the difficulty distinguishing between
                    small-for-dates and premature fetuses. If menstrual
                    dates were indeed reliable there would be no
                    problem.

Ref 15

1.187 The incidence of the following conditions is increased in a growth retarded neonate:
A idiopathic respiratory distress syndrome
B pulmonary haemorrhage
C meconium aspiration syndrome
D hypoglycaemia
E anaemia

1.188 The following factors are associated with fetal growth retardation:
A intra uterine infection
B teenage pregnancy
C pregnancy at high altitude
D post oral contraception pregnancy
E heroin addiction

1.189 Turner's syndrome
A is associated with neonatal oedema of the feet
B babies display neonatal sneezing
C is the commonest chromosomal abnormality in aborted fetuses
D has ventricular septal defect as the commonest cardiac abnormality
E is autosomal dominant

1.190 Mental retardation is associated with
A cystic fibrosis
B congenital Toxoplasmosis
C XXX genotype
D fetal alcohol syndrome
E gonadal dysgenesis

1.191 Transplacental infection occurs with
A echo virus
B malaria
C rubella
D syphilis
E gonorrhoea

(*Answers overleaf*)

1.187 A **False**   The growth retarded neonate is exposed to many
  B **True**   hazards, but these do not include the idiopathic
  C **True**   respiratory distress syndrome unless it is also
  D **True**   premature. A growth retarded baby is more prone to
  E **False**   intra partum asphyxia and consequently pulmonary
   haemorrhage. Meconium aspiration may result from
   asphyxia. Reduced glycogen stores predispose to
   hypoglycaemia and these neonates are more likely to
   be polycythaemic.

Ref 15

1.188 A **True**   Fetal growth retardation is of two types; symmetrical
  B **True**   and asymmetrical. If an insult occurs early or
  C **True**   throughout pregnancy then growth retardation tends
  D **False**   to be symmetrical with both head and body reduced
  E **True**   in size. This occurs in congenital disorders, intra
   uterine infection or drug abuse. If the event occurs
   later, as in pre eclampsia, then the abdomen stops
   growing before the head in an asymmetrical fashion.
   Small women have small babies, as do women living
   at high altitude and there is an unexpected high
   incidence of IUGR in young teenagers.

Ref 16

1.189 A **True**   Turner's syndrome, usually of XO genotype, is the
  B **False**   commonest chromosomal abnormality in abnormal
  C **True**   fetuses. If the child is born alive they have streak
  D **False**   gonads, sometimes have oedema of the feet and the
  E **False**   commonest cardiac abnormality is coarctation of the
   aorta. Sneezing occurs with maternal heroin
   addiction.

Ref 16

1.190 A **False**   Congenital toxoplasmosis causes convulsions,
  B **True**   hydrocephaly, spastic paralysis and mental
  C **True**   retardation. Mental retardation is also one of the
  D **True**   features of the fetal alcohol syndrome. Mental
  E **False**   retardation and menstrual abnormalities are features
   of XXX female but they may be normal

D Harvey & I Kovacs in Ref 3

1.191 A **True**   In years gone by syphilis was a very common cause
  B **True**   of intra-uterine death or congenital neonatal
  C **True**   infection. The echo and Coxackie viruses as well as
  D **True**   the TORCH infections (including rubella) are now
  E **False**   regarded as important causes of congenital
   abnormality following transplacental infection.

I Kovacs & D Harvey in Ref 3

1.192 Congenital syphilis causes
A a neonatal rash
B raised cord blood IgM
C blindness
D abnormal facies
E abnormal teeth

1.193 The following organisms are transmitted from mother to baby during delivery
A toxoplasma gondii
B hepatitis B virus
C herpes hominis, type I
D chlamydia
E streptococcus pyogenes, Lancefield group B

1.194 ABO erythroblastosis fetalis
A is less common then rhesus erythroblastosis fetalis
B occurs principally in the first born infant
C becomes more severe with subsequent pregnancies
D occurs in Group O infants born to Group A or B mothers
E causes jaundice earlier than in rhesus incompatibility

1.195 Alpha-feto protein
A accounts for 25% of fetal globulins at the end of the first trimester
B has a maximal concentration in fetal serum at 12–14 weeks
C has a maximal concentration in maternal serum at 20 weeks
D in the maternal serum shows no correlation with amniotic fluid levels in normal pregnancy
E maternal serum alpha-feto protein measurements fall with abortion induced by intra-amniotic prostaglandins, or urea

(Answers overleaf)

1.192 A **True**   Congenital syphilis manifests in many ways but a
     B **True**   fetus at risk should have cord blood taken for
     C **True**   Immunoglobilin level for diagnosis. All of the above
     D **True**   features are recognized but especially facial
     E **True**   disfigurement with a saddle nose and notch shaped
     (Hutchinsons) teeth. Corneal scarring due to
     interstitial keratitis causes defective vision.

Ref 16

1.193 A **False**   Toxoplasmosis and other TORCH infections produce
     B **True**   antepartum infection of the neonate Hepatitis B,
     C **False**   Herpes type II, Chlamydia and pyogenic organisms
     D **True**   including the gonococcus may infect the fetus during
     E **True**   delivery. Caesarean section may be indicated in order
     to avoid neonatal herpes viraemia.

Ref 16

1.194 A **False**   Although ABO erythroblastosis is more common
     B **True**   than that due to rhesus incompatibility the disease is
     C **False**   less severe with the cord blood haemoglobin rarely
     D **False**   decreased and exchange transfusion rarely required.
     E **False**   It is more insidious and problems of haemolysis
     occur later then in rhesus disease. Unlike rhesus
     iso-immunization it usually affects the first born and
     does not become worse in subsequent pregnancies.
     It appears almost exclusively in Group A or B infants
     born to Group O mothers.

Ref 16

1.195 A **True**   Alpha-feto protein has a molecular weight the same
     B **True**   as albumen — i.e. 69 000 and accounts for 25% of
     C **False**   fetal globulins at the end of the first trimester. It is
     D **True**   often known as the fetal albumen, has a maximal
     E **False**   concentration in the fetus at 12–14 weeks and in the
     mother at 36 weeks which shows no correlation with
     amniotic fluid levels in normal pregnancy. Maternal
     serum AFP levels increase with induced
     mid-trimester abortion.

M J Bennett in Ref 3 Vol 1

1.196 Elevated maternal serum alpha-feto protein levels in the second trimester are characteristically found with
A incorrect gestational age
B diabetes mellitus
C intrauterine death
D threatened abortion
E hydatidiform mole

1.197 Human placental lactogen (HPL) would be expected to be low in
A diabetic pregnancy
B sensitized Rhesus negative pregnancy at an early stage
C pregnancy at 44 weeks' gestation
D anencephalic fetus
E multiple pregnancy

1.198 The following affect urinary oestriol levels in a pregnant woman:
A Mandelamine
B Ampicillin
C Betamethasone
D placental sulphatase deficiency
E Trimethoprim

1.199 The following are major indicators of fetal asphyxia
A fresh meconium at induction of labour
B loss of beat to beat variation
C deep type I dips in the second stage of labour
D type II dips with basal tachycardia
E excessive fetal movements

1.200 Intra partum fetal blood sampling
A should be performed following second stage type II dips
B is useful in Rhesus disease
C reduces the Caesarean section rate in monitored patients
D is used to measure fetal pO_2
E can be used to assess diabetic control

(*Answers overleaf*)

1.196 A **True**   It is possible that maternal AFP assays would be
       B **False**   more helpful in detection of high risk pregnancies
       C **True**   following mid-trimester bleeds, twins and fetal
       D **True**   growth retardation than in the detection of neural
       E **False**   tube defects as these can be picked up in skilled
                     hands by ultra-sound. Ultra-sonic dating between
                     16–18 weeks is essential when interpreting these
                     results.

M J Bennett in Ref 3 Vol 1

1.197 A **False**   HPL is produced by the trophoblast and reflects
       B **False**   placental size reasonably well. Multiple pregnancies,
       C **True**   diabetic pregnancies and affected Rhesus negative
       D **False**   pregnancies have large placentas and raised levels.
       E **False**   HPL levels are normal in pregnancies with an
                     abnormal fetus. HPL level is no longer regarded as a
                     useful placental function test.

W N Spellacy in Ref 5

1.198 A **False**   Oestriol production by the fetoplacental unit depends
       B **True**   on intact adrenal and placental function. Ampicillin
       C **True**   interferes with the entero hepatic circulation of
       D **True**   oestrogen metabolites, betamethasone suppresses
       E **False**   adrenal function and placental sulphatase is part of
                     the enzyme pathway. Multiple pregnancy is also
                     associated with elevated oestriols.

1.199 A **True**   This is a difficult question of interpretation of these
       B **False**   events. Type II dips with tachycardia is the clearest
       C **False**   abnormality. Most would accept that fresh meconium
       D **True**   at induction is an important warning sign but loss of
       E **False**   beat to beat variation is more often due to drugs or
                     fetal sleep. Type I second stage deceleration are so
                     common as to be almost regarded as normal. The
                     significance of excessive fetal movements is doubtful
                     but some convulsive movements may be associated
                     with acute asphyxia.

J Pearson in Ref 3 Vol 1

1.200 A **False**   Fetal blood sampling is used to assess fetal asphyxia
       B **True**   but second stage type II dips are an indication for
       C **True**   delivery. It can be used for monitoring blood glucose
       D **False**   levels in diabetics, and haemoglobin, blood group
       E **True**   and Coomb's test in Rhesus disease.

Ref 'various'

1.201 Immunoglobulins
A are alpha globulins
B of the G group cross the placenta
C of the M group do not cross the placenta
D are used for active immunization
E are useful in the neonate for confirmation of intra-uterine infection

1.202 A patient at 34 weeks with premature membrane rupture who is not in labour should
A receive prophylactic antibiotics
B receive betamethazone
C receive tocolytic drugs if contractions occur
D have a vaginal and cervical swab taken for culture
E not have a vaginal examination digitally

1.203 Chorioamnionitis
A is caused by listeria monocytogenes
B is more common in premature labours
C causes amniorrhexis
D is rarely due to N Gonorrhoea
E is treated with corticosteroids

1.204 Amniotic fluid infection is prevented by
A the placenta
B IgM
C IgG
D meconium
E the cervical mucus plug

(*Answers overleaf*)

1.201 A **False**   Immunoglobulins are part of the gamma globulin
    B **True**   fraction. Immunoglobulins of the G group (IgG) cross
    C **True**   the placenta and confer passive immunity of a
    D **False**   temporary nature on the neonate. M group
    E **True**   molecules (IgM) do not cross the placenta and if
found in cord blood or neonatal blood confirm that
intra-uterine infection has occurred. Passive
immunization of a short term nature is conferred by
immunoglobulin injections. Active immunization
requires attenuated or killed virus and confers longer
term immunity.

Ref 16

1.202 A **False**   This patient needs to be delivered as a survival at 34
    B **False**   weeks should be in excess of 96%. The patient should
    C **False**   have a sterile speculum examination to confirm the
    D **True**   diagnosis, and swabs are probably relevant.
    E **True**   Prophylactic antibiotics and betamethazone are
contra indicated. Betamethazone is of doubtful value
at 34 weeks and increases the risk of infection.

K Ritchie, G McClure in Ref 3 Vol 2

1.203 A **True**   Chorioamnionitis is caused by aerobic and anaerobic
    B **True**   vaginal flora, but N gonorrhoea is the most common
    C **True**   exogenous organism and listeria monocytogenes the
    D **False**   most classical example of infection with intact
    E **False**   membranes. Low grade chorioamnionitis is probably
a very common cause of spontaneous pre-term
membrane rupture. Treatment consists of
intramuscular antibiotics and delivery

R Schwartz in Ref 3 Vol 2

1.204 A **False**   The host defences are (1) anatomical barriers of skin,
    B **False**   membranes and mucus plug but not the placenta; (2)
    C **True**   innate immunity and (3) specific immune response
    D **False**   through IgG and cell mediated immunity. Meconium
    E **True**   staining, prematurity and malnutrition remove the
bacteriocidal qualities of amniotic fluid.

R Schwartz in Ref 3 Vol 2

1.205 Human fetal breathing movements
A do not occur until the third trimester of pregnancy
B may be absent for one hour in normal pregnancy
C show a significant variation in incidence over a 24 hour period
D are increased in diabetic pregnancies
E are a reliable indicator of fetal hypoxia

1.206 Ultrasound is useful in making the following fetal diagnoses:
A spina bifida
B Down's syndrome
C Turner's syndrome
D oesophageal atresia
E osteogenesis imperfecta

1.207 Fetal trunk movements in the third trimester
A are increased by administration of glucose to the mother
B are less frequent towards term
C are less well perceived by primigravid patients
D are generally reduced in the hypoxic fetus
E usually stop at least 12 hours before fetal death due to chronic hypoxia

(*Answers overleaf*)

1.205 A **False**   Fetal breathing movements may be observed
B **True**   ultrasonically from early in the second trimester. In
C **True**   the third trimester they occur for about 40% of the
D **True**   time and show a marked diurnal variation. Their
E **False**   occurrence is highly episodic and in normal
pregnancy periods of apnoea of over 2 hours have
been observed. Thus, short observation periods (30
minutes) are unreliable in the diagnosis of fetal
hypoxia. The incidence of breathing correlates
positively with blood glucose concentration and is
increased in diabetic pregnancy.

S Campbell, D Griffin in Ref 3 Vol 3

1.206 A **True**   Ultrasonic examination is useful in the diagnosis of
B **False**   any fetal anomaly that is characterized by anatomical
C **True**   deformity (e.g. spina bifida, exomphalos, dwarfism)
D **True**   or obstruction in a hollow viscus (duodenal atresia,
E **True**   obstructive uropathy). Anomalies showing no gross
anatomical defect, such as Down's syndrome, may
not be diagnosed at present except indirectly via
other associated defects (duodenal atresia,
congenital heart disease). Shortening of limbs,
reduced calcification and intra-uterine fractures in
osteogenesis imperfect gravis can be recognized
ultrasonically.

S Campbell, D Griffin in Ref 3 Vol 3

1.207 A **False**   Fetal trunk movements occur for about 20% of the
B **True**   time during the third trimester. Unlike fetal breathing
C **False**   movements, they are not affected by administration
D **True**   of glucose to the mother. The maternal perception of
E **True**   movements is dependent only upon the number of
fetal parts moving and independent of parity,
gestational age, obesity, etc. Although widely
variable in incidence, fetal movements are generally
reduced in the hypoxic fetus and will usually stop at
least 12 hours before fetal death.

S Campbell, D Griffin in Ref 3 Vol 3

1.208 The following statements are true about ultrasonic examination:

A biparietal diameter measurement will indicate fetal post-menstrual age to ± one week from 12 to 32 weeks

B the abdominal circumference has a better correlation with fetal weight than the biparietal diameter

C the head circumference to abdomen circumference ratio is depressed in the macrosomic fetus

D the finding of a placenta that covers the internal os at 30 weeks menstrual age will necessitate eventual delivery by elective Caesarean section

E duodenal atresia is associated with the 'triple bubble'

(*Answers overleaf*)

1.208 A **False**   Ultrasonic biparietal measurement is only accurate in
    B **True**   assessing the post menstrual age of the fetus until
    C **True**   the 26th post menstrual week. Thereafter, varying
    D **False**   fetal growth rates make dating less accurate. The
    E **False**   abdomen circumference measurement reflects fetal
liver size and correlates well with somatic growth and
fetal weight. Head circumference measurement
reflects brain growth which is less affected by factors
influencing growth. Thus, the macrosomic infant will
exhibit a low head circumference to abdomen
circumference ratio whereas an asymetrically
growth retarded fetus will have a high ratio. Elective
Caesarean section should not be performed on the
basis of placental localization, performed more than
two weeks prior to delivery. The fetus with duodenal
atresia has a 'double bubble' of dilated duodenum
and stomach separated by the pylorus.

S Campbell, D Griffin in Ref 3 Vol 3

2. Gynaecology

2.1 Endometriosis
A is more common in white patients than black
B contains struma ovarii
C characteristically occurs in nulliparous patients
D causes cyclical pneumothoraces
E is best diagnosed by laparoscopy in the follicular phase

2.2 Hydatidiform mole
A usually has female chromosomes
B arises from the amnion
C typically shows avascularity of the trophoblastic villi
D secretes luteinizing hormone
E shows trophoblastic proliferation

2.3 Hydatidiform mole
A occurs more commonly in West Africa than in the United Kingdom
B shows a snow storm appearance on ultrasonic examination
C can be diagnosed by chest X-ray
D commonly presents with vaginal bleeding
E is followed by choriocarcinoma in 25% of cases in the United Kingdom

2.4 Hydatidiform moles
A occur more commonly in women of blood group A married to blood group 0 men
B are commoner in older gravidae
C are complicated by thyrotoxicosis
D are complicated by ovarian cysts
E less frequently cause malignancies if husband and wife's blood group is the same

(*Answers overleaf*)

2.1 A **True**   Endometriosis occurs most commonly in females of
     B **False**   low parity but not necessarily without children. It is
     C **False**   characteristically rare in black patients, but this
     D **True**   difference is becoming less marked. Ectopic
     E **False**   endometrium may occur in any site and is recorded
                     in the lungs and pleura. The timing of laparoscopy,
                     especially in serial assessment is important as black
                     spots are most apparent before or during
                     menstruation.

G Schneider in Ref 3 Vol 3

2.2 A **True**   Hydatidiform mole, in the majority of cases having a
     B **False**   female chromosome complement, arises from the
     C **True**   trophoblast. The pathological changes
     D **False**   characteristically show trophoblastic proliferation,
     E **True**   hydropic degeneration of the villus and scantiness of
                     the blood vessels. Helpful in diagnosis is its secretion
                     of human chorionic gonadotrophin (HCG)
                     antigenically similar to luteinizing hormone (LH).

J S Scott in Ref 4

2.3 A **True**   There is a clear geographical variation in incidence of
     B **True**   hydatidiform mole with more cases in the Far East
     C **False**   and Africa. A snow storm appearance on ultrasonic
     D **True**   examination is diagnostic. An abnormal chest X-ray
     E **False**   is very uncommon, but may occur with metastasizing
                     mole or choriocarcinoma. Most cases of mole
                     present with vaginal bleeding as a threatened
                     abortion. Choriocarcinoma follows mole in 1–20% of
                     cases but in the United Kingdom the lower figure is
                     more likely on account of careful follow up and
                     treatment of persistent moles as well as less
                     malignant potential.

J S Scott in Ref 4

2.4 A **True**   Group A women married to Group O men have a ten
     B **True**   times greater risk than A–A partnerships. Group AB
     C **True**   women have the worst prognosis. More than 10% of
     D **True**   patients have thyrotoxicosis due to the production of
     E **True**   molar thyrotrophin and 15% develop bilateral
                     theca-lutein cysts due to excessive HCG secretion.

J S Scott in Ref 4

2.5   The benign lesions associated with DES exposure include
   A   oligospermia in males
   B   Cocks-comb appearance in males
   C   cervical hoods
   D   vaginal location of the squamo-columnar junction
   E   uterine hyperplasia

2.6   Uterine fibroids
   A   are more common in black patients
   B   are associated with nulliparity
   C   characteristically cause pain
   D   should be removed at Caesarean section if larger than 2 cm
       diameter
   E   undergo sarcomatous change in 1% of cases

2.7   Red degeneration of a uterine fibroid
   A   only occurs in pregnancy
   B   causes a leucopaenia with a lymphocytosis
   C   is associated with a raised ESR
   D   is aseptic infarction
   E   is due to emboli occluding the major blood vessels supplying
       the myoma.

2.8   Uterine fibroids
   A   are primarily composed of fibrous tissue
   B   characteristically present with intermenstrual bleeding
   C   may be seen on a plain abdominal X-ray
   D   are associated with endometriosis
   E   have a capsule

(*Answers overleaf*)

2.5   A **True**   DES exposure in utero in males may produce
      B **False**   oligospermia, hypospadias and epididymal cysts. In
      C **True**   the female, the benign changes are vaginal adenosis,
      D **True**   cervical hoods, ridges and cocks – combs and also
      E **False**   uterine hypoplasia. There is often a vaginal location
                      of the squamo-columnar junction and colposcopic
                      follow-up of these lesions is required.

S J Robboy in Ref 3 Vol 1

2.6   A **True**   Fibroids are more common in women of negro origin
      B **True**   and associated with nulliparity and infertility
      C **False**   although less so in black patients. Fibroids are often
      D **False**   asymptomatic and do not cause pain unless they
      E **False**   twist, undergo malignant change or co-exist with
                      sepsis and endometriosis. Fibroids should not be
                      removed at Caesarean section because of the risk of
                      haemorrhage. They undergo sarcomatous change in
                      less than 0.5% of cases.

R M Feroze in Ref 4

2.7   A **False**   Red degeneration can also occur in non-pregnant
      B **False**   women generally over the age of 40 if the fibroids are
      C **True**   large. The patient has a generalized leucocytosis, is
      D **True**   febrile and has a raised ESR. The condition is due to
      E **False**   the tumour outgrowing its own blood supply and
                      leading to an aseptic degeneration and infarction.
                      Histologically venous thrombosis are present but this
                      is not due to embolic episodes.

Ref 6

2.8   A **False**   Uterine fibroids or myomata consist of bundles of
      B **False**   smooth muscle which develop more fibrous tissue as
      C **True**   they grow larger. They present with menorrhagia,
      D **True**   usually without dysmenorrhea but do not
      E **False**   characteristically produce intermenstrual bleeding.
                      Large fibroids may appear as soft tissue masses on
                      X-ray and calcified fibroids are readily visible. 60% of
                      myomata occur in women with one or no
                      pregnancies. They do not have a true capsule.

R M Feroze in Ref 4

2.9   Dysfunctional uterine bleeding is associated with
   A chronic pelvic inflammatory disease
   B abnormal hormone profiles in more than 50% of patients
   C increased levels of PGE_2 in the endometrium
   D oestrogens inhibiting the arachidonic acid cascade
   E metropathia haemorrhagica

2.10   The following have been shown to be effective in the treatment of dysfunctional uterine bleeding:
   A tranexamic acid
   B methyl testosterone
   C neostigmine bromide
   D clomiphene
   E epsilon amino caproic acid.

2.11   The following are associated with dysfunctional uterine bleeding:
   A hypothyroidism
   B Von Willebrand's disease
   C subserous fibroids
   D afibrinogenaemia
   E thrombocytopaenic purpura

2.12   A suspicion of pregnancy of eight weeks gestation may be confirmed by
   A vaginal examination
   B abdominal examination
   C breast examination
   D an immunological pregnancy test
   E an ultrasonic scan

(Answers overleaf)

2.9   A **False**   Dysfunctional uterine bleeding is heavy uterine
      B **False**   bleeding in the absence of tumour, infection or
      C **True**   pregnancy and by definition is not due to chronic
      D **False**   sepsis. It is unusual to find abnormal hormone
      E **True**   profiles and although anovulation and metropathia
                        are well-defined pictures, they only occur in a small
                        minority of cases. Oestrogens enhance and
                        progestogens inhibit the arachidonic acid cascade
                        which probably initiates menstruation.

D A Davey in Ref 4

2.10 A **True**   19-Nortestosterone derivatives (Norethisterone) are
      B **True**   primarily used as hormone therapy for dysfunctional
      C **False**   uterine bleeding. Androgens have been used
      D **True**   successfully and the anti-fibrinolytics amino caproic
      E **True**   acid and tranexamic acid have been shown to be
                        effective. Clomiphene, although not ideal because of
                        side effects, is also effective when the dysfunctional
                        uterine bleeding is anovulatory.

D A Davey in Ref 4

2.11 A **True**   Dysfunctional uterine bleeding is associated with
      B **True**   thyroid dysfunction especially hypothyroidism.
      C **False**   Excessive bleeding is common in Von Willebrand's
      D **False**   disease and thrombocytopaenic purpura but not in
      E **True**   afibrinogenaemia, hypothrombinaemia and heparin
                        therapy. Anticoagulation does not cause
                        menorrhagia. The clotting system does not seem to
                        be important.

D A Davey in Ref 4

2.12 A **False**   Vaginal examination may reveal signs of
      B **False**   oestrogenisation, softening and change of shape of
      C **False**   the uterus but is not reliable enough to confirm
      D **True**   pregnancy. Breast examination may reveal
      E **True**   enlargement, pigmentation of the areola,
                        Montgomery's tubercles or expression of fluid from
                        the nipple but these signs are not enough to confirm
                        pregnancy. An immunological pregnancy test or
                        ultrasonic scan should confirm the diagnosis at this
                        stage.

Ref 6

2.13 Dermoid cysts
A   are germ cell tumours
B   are bilateral in 40–60% of cases
C   are the commonest cysts detected during pregnancy
D   are malignant in 10% of cases
E   are frequently XY

2.14 In Meig's syndrome
A   the hydrothorax is composed of peritoneal fluid
B   the hydrothorax occurs most commonly on the left side
C   the ovarian lesion may be a Brenner tumour
D   the hyrothorax requires chemotherapy
E   the fibroma is frequently more than 10 cm in size

2.15 Theca lutein cysts
A   are bilateral
B   develop in normal pregnancy
C   may be iatrogenic
D   excrete human chorionic gonadotrophin
E   require surgical removal

2.16 The International Society for the Study of Vulval Disease (1973) made the following recommendations:
A   Bowen's Disease remains as a separate entity
B   Hyperplastic dystrophy includes leucoplakia
C   Hypoplastic dystrophy with atypia is a suggested term
D   Carcinoma in situ is not a useful diagnosis
E   Kraurosis is included in the term hypoplastic dystrophy

2.17 The following should be treated by simple vulvectomy:
A   Melanoma
B   Paget's disease
C   vulval carcinoma in situ
D   intractable pruritus vulvae in older patients
E   herpes

(*Answers overleaf*)

2.13 A **True**   Ovarian teratomas are practically always XX.
     B **False**   Dermoid cysts occur in young women and are
     C **True**   bilateral in 10–12% of cases. As they occur in this
     D **False**   age group they are common in pregnancy and the
     E **False**   'weight' of the semi solid cyst encourages the
                     formation of a pedicle and torsion. They are
                     malignant in less than 5% of cases.

Ref 20

2.14 A **True**   The solid fibroma which characteristically produces
     B **False**   Meig's syndrome of ascites and hydrothorax is
     C **True**   usually small. The syndrome has also been described
     D **False**   with Brenner tumour, granulosa cell tumour and
     E **False**   thecoma. This syndrome was first described by
                     Lawson Tait at the end of the 19th Century.

Ref 20

2.15 A **True**   Theca lutein cysts are large bilateral polycystic
     B **True**   masses which rarely occur in normal pregnancy but
     C **True**   frequently with trophoblastic disease due to excess
     D **False**   gonadotrophin secretion and with hyperstimulation
     E **False**   with gonadotrophins. They regress spontaneously
                     and do not require surgical removal.

Ref 20

2.16 A **False**   The suggested terms were (1) hypoplastic dystrophy,
     B **True**   (2) hyperplastic dystrophy with or without atypia and
     C **False**   (3) mixed dystrophy with or without atypia.
     D **False**   Carcinoma in situ and Paget's disease are regarded
     E **True**   as intra-epithelial neoplasia. Apart from Paget's
                     disease, no other eponymous terms should be used.

C Douglas in Ref 3 Vol 3

2.17 A **False**   Paget's disease of the vulva and carcinoma in situ
     B **True**   should certainly be treated by no more than a simple
     C **True**   vulvectomy. Melanoma with node involvement has a
     D **True**   bad prognosis and although secondaries are both
     E **False**   lymph and blood-borne it is strongly recommended
                     that radical vulvectomy with inguinal and iliac
                     lymphadenectomy is indicated. Intractable
                     pruritis vulvae is perhaps more contentious, but if in
                     the older age group the irritation is, as the question
                     states, intractable, vulvectomy usually gives more
                     than temporary relief.

Ref 12

2.18 The following statements about vulval ulceration are true:
    A granuloma venereum can be diagnosed by finding Donovan bodies
    B lymphogranuloma venereum has a viral aetiology
    C tetracycline is effective in treating both granuloma and lymphogranuloma venereum
    D Behcet's syndrome has a immunological aetiology
    E Behcet's ulcers are pre-malignant

2.19 Ultrasonic examination has a certain place in the diagnosis of the following gynaecological problems:
    A endometrial carcinoma
    B Asherman's syndrome
    C ascites
    D ovulation
    E uterine septum

2.20 In pelvic endometriosis
    A the amount of pelvic pain is related to the extent of the disease
    B there is a close association with the unruptured follicle syndrome
    C the tubes are rarely blocked
    D clomid should be used to induce ovulation
    E treatment by Danazol may produce hirsutism

2.21 The following would be first choice antibiotic therapy:
    A Clindamycin for bacteroides
    B Streptomycin and pasinah for pelvic tuberculosis
    C Procaine penicillin for syphilis
    D Ampicillin for prophylaxis against gonorrhoea
    E Ampicillin and gentamycin as prophylaxis during delivery for patients with heart disease

2.22 Pelvic actinomycosis
    A is due to a gram negative fungus
    B is usually right sided
    C is treated with Streptomycin
    D may follow the colonisation of the uterus which occurs in 5% of plastic IUCD users
    E produces fistulae

(*Answers overleaf*)

2.18   A **True**   The aetiology of Behcet's syndrome is quite
       B **True**   unknown, but it has not, like granuloma venereum, a
       C **True**   malignant potential. Tetracycline is the best antibiotic
       D **False**   for both the bacterial granuloma and the viral
       E **False**   lympho-granuloma. The diagnosis is made by finding
                         Donovan bodies and a positive Frei test respectively.

C J Dewhurst in Ref 4

2.19   A **False**   In gynaecology ultrasound has proven useful in the
       B **False**   diagnosis of early pregnancy complications,
       C **True**   abnormal uterine shape, hydatidiform mole,
       D **True**   diagnosis of ovulation and the recognition of ovarian
       E **True**   masses or ascites.

2.20   A **False**   Pain is often most severe in minimal 'black spot'
       B **True**   disease. Although infertile, the patient's tubes are
       C **True**   rarely blocked. There is a suggestion that the
       D **False**   peritoneal fluid hormone concentrations present
       E **True**   when the follicle fails to rupture does not inhibit
                         endometrial seedling growth, and therefore may be
                         an aetiological factor in this condition. Clomid does
                         not help and Danazol produces a
                         pseudo-menopausal state with symptoms of hot
                         flushes, hirsutism and acne.

G Schneider in Ref 3 Vol 3

2.21   A **False**   Members of our specialty are unwilling to use
       B **False**   antibiotics such as gentamycin and kanamycin which
       C **True**   with the correct safeguards are effective and safe
       D **False**   antibiotics. Clindamycin seems to be preferred
       E **True**   although the complication of necrotising enteritis is a
                         fatal one. A single injection of 80 mg gentamycin and
                         two days of ampicillin is the ideal prophylaxis against
                         subacute bacterial endocarditis in patients at risk.
                         There is no effective prophylactic antibiotic against
                         the increasingly resistant gonococcus.

Ref 'various'

2.22   A **False**   A. israeli is a gram positive mycelium forming fungus
       B **True**   which usually has its origins in the appendix. Cervical
       C **False**   colonisation by actinomycosis occurs in 30% of
       D **False**   women with plastic devices and less than 2% with
       E **True**   copper-containing devices. Chronic tubo-ovarian
                         abscesses and fistulae occur and the treatment is by
                         high dose penicillin.

Ref 20

2.23 Pelvic tuberculosis
 A   is most often bovine
 B   is post primary
 C   is associated with amenorrhoea
 D   more often involves the fallopian tubes than endometrium
 E   is decreasing in the United Kingdom

2.24 The following statements regarding anti-tuberculous chemotherapy for pelvic disease are correct:
 A   streptomycin is first line therapy
 B   chemotherapy is continued for eighteen months
 C   isoniazid causes peripheral neuropathy, treatable by Pyridoxine
 D   ethambutol causes blindness
 E   chemotherapy should not be commenced if histology is positive and the culture is negative

2.25 Actinomycosis
 A   is associated with Toxic Shock syndrome
 B   can be recognized by cervical cytology
 C   occurs with a Lippes loop IUD
 D   spreads from the appendix
 E   is best treated by intra-muscular penicillin

2.26 A surgical approach to a pelvic abscess is indicated
 A   if a tubo-ovarian abscess ruptures
 B   if the abscess is sub-acute
 C   if the diagnosis is in doubt
 D   if the patient is sensitive to penicillin
 E   if a mass is present after seven days of effective antibiotic therapy

(Answers overleaf)

2.23 A **False**   Pelvic tuberculosis is nearly always of human type,
     B **True**   although rare vulval lesion may be of bovine type.
     C **True**   Infection becomes apparent after puberty and years
     D **True**   after the primary lesion has healed. Menorrhagia,
     E **False**   pain, infertility and also amenorrhoea are features.
                    The fallopian tube is involved in 100% of cases and
                    the endometrium in 80%. The incidence of
                    tuberculosis is increasing now, following
                    immigration.

C R Whitfield in Ref 4

2.24 A **False**   First choice treatment for tuberculosis is Rifampicin
     B **False**   and Isoniazid and/or Ethambutol. It should continue
     C **True**   for eight to twelve months and will often be
     D **True**   prescribed before positive cultures are available (they
     E **False**   may be negative). These drugs have very severe side
                    effects, including retro-bulbar neuritis (Ethambutol),
                    8th cranial nerve damage (Streptomycin) and
                    peripheral neuropathy (Isoniazid)

Ref 'various'

2.25 A **False**   Actinomycosis is a chronic infection which may
     B **True**   spread from the gut, particularly the appendix, and is
     C **True**   now found in patients with a plastic intra-uterine
     D **True**   device. Treatment is by a long course of
     E **True**   intra-muscular penicillin. Toxic shock syndrome is
                    associated with high absorbency tampons which are
                    left in the vagina for several days during
                    menstruation.

Ref 20

2.26 A **True**   Surgery is necessary if an abscess ruptures, if the
     B **False**   diagnosis is in doubt or if there is no response to
     C **True**   antibiotics. Post partum pelvic abscess more
     D **False**   commonly requires surgical drainage. If the mass is
     E **False**   smaller within seven days surgery can be withheld as
                    there are particular dangers of bowel injury if surgery
                    is performed on a responding sub-acute abscess.

I Brown in Ref 3 Vol 2

2.27 The following general surgical statements are true:
A Catgut should not be used for the ovarian capsular closure after wedge resection.
B Elective appendicectomy is justified at the same time as ovarian or tubal surgery.
C One should attempt to save the affected tube when dealing with an ectopic pregnancy.
D Suturing the cardinal ligaments at vaginal hysterectomy prevent a post operative enterocoele.
E The ovaries should generally be removed at abdominal hysterectomy after the age of 40 years.

2.28 At the time of abdominal hysterectomy the ureters may be characteristically damaged at:
A vaginal vault
B the broad ligaments
C the resuturing of the parietal peritoneum
D the division of the infundibular pelvic ligament
E removal of co-existent parovarian cyst

2.29 A vaginal hysterectomy
A should not be performed if there is no uterine descent
B should only be performed if the uterus is of normal size
C should not be performed if there is cervical intra-epithelial neoplasia
D needs a routine post-operative indwelling catheter
E may be complicated by a post-operative rectocele

2.30 The following are long-term problems that occur after hysterectomy and bilateral oophorectomy:
A depression
B enterocoele
C hysteria
D headaches
E fatigue

(Answers overleaf)

2.27 A **True**   The use of catgut in the ovary or unnecessary
     B **False**   appendicectomy at this time are two important ways
     C **True**   of producing fimbrial adhesions and infertility.
     D **False**   Current surgical views are that the tube and ovary
     E **False**   should be conserved in the examples given, although
                     the risk of an ectopic and the increasing incidence of
                     ovarian cancer may change these views in the future
                     in favour of willing sub-fertility and oestrogen
                     therapy respectively. The utero-sacral ligaments are
                     approximated in order to prevent enterocoele.

2.28 A **True**   The ureters are characteristically damaged by the
     B **True**   inexperienced or the unlucky if the pelvic ligaments
     C **False**   or the uterine vessels or the uterine angle are
     D **True**   clamped too far laterally, or as a result of
     E **True**   haemostasis during a difficult procedure. The
                     posterior leaf of the broad ligament is also a
                     danger-area particularly with broad ligament fibroids,
                     endometriosis or a para-ovarian cyst. Even when the
                     uterus has been removed the closure of the visceral
                     peritoneum is a time when the ureters may be
                     included in the suture.

Ref 22

2.29 A **False**   In general the vaginal route is the ideal way of
     B **False**   performing a hysterectomy as there are fewer
     C **False**   post-operative complications. Vaginal hysterectomy
     D **False**   can be performed without a pelvic floor repair if there
     E **False**   is no descent. Neither moderate enlargement nor CIN
                     lesions are an obstacle to this operation.
                     Post-operative catheterisation is not required if there
                     is no anterior repair. A possible complication is an
                     enterocele.

Ref 22

2.30 A **True**   It is difficult to be sure whether a post-hysterectomy
     B **False**   syndrome occurs if the ovaries are conserved.
     C **False**   However, bilateral oophorectomy produces hot
     D **True**   flushes, sweats, headaches, irritability, depression,
     E **True**   fatigue and sexual problems. Others would claim that
                     these sort of problems would occur even after an
                     umcomplicated hysterectomy, but it is likely that
                     there would have been a preceding affective
                     disorder.

Ref 22

2.31 The following are helpful in the diagnosis of syphilis
   A   CFT
   B   FTA
   C   VDRL
   D   gram stain
   E   examination of contact

2.32 Acute salpingitis
   A   occurs in approximately 40% of patients with untreated
       endocervical gonorrhoea
   B   is more often caused by non-gonococcal infection than by
       gonorrhoea
   C   rarely has unilateral symptoms
   D   may be excluded if the pregnancy test is positive
   E   should be treated with an oral penicillin and Probenecid

2.33 An acute exacerbation of chronic pelvic inflammatory disease
   A   occurs characteristically after menstruation
   B   is caused by mycoplasma
   C   is treated with guidance from high vaginal swab bacteriology
       results
   D   should be treated on an in-patient basis
   E   needs parenteral therapy

**2.34 The following are characteristic symptoms of chronic pelvic
inflammatory disease:**
   A   vaginal dryness
   B   irregular menstruation
   C   Backache
   D   fever
   E   constipation

2.35 Genuine stress incontinence in the female
   A   occurs transiently during pregnancy
   B   is more common in parous women
   C   is corrected surgically
   D   is associated with a low urethral pressure profile amplitude
       on urodynamic studies
   E   is not always associated with utero-vaginal prolapse

(*Answers overleaf*)

2.31 A **False**   The certain diagnosis of syphilis can be difficult and
      B **True**   the FTA test is the most reliable. The VDRL is very
      C **True**   non-specific, picking up yaws and malaria. A gram
      D **False**   stain is useless and putting any reliability on the
      E **False**   examination of a contact assumes a monogamous
                    relationship.

2.32 A **False**   Salpingitis is most commonly caused by
      B **True**   non-gonococcal infection and occurs in 10%–20% of
      C **False**   patients with a positive endocervical culture for
      D **False**   gonorrhoea. Symptoms are often unilateral although
      E **False**   bilateral pain is more common. Treatment should be
                    by parenteral antibiotics in order to minimize the risk
                    of subsequent tubal damage.

Ref 12

2.33 A **True**   Exacerbations of pelvic inflammatory disease occur
      B **True**   after menstruation. It is now thought to be commonly
      C **False**   caused by mycoplasma organisms. The taking of a
      D **True**   high vaginal swab although traditional will rarely
      E **True**   reveal organisms which are pathogenic and it
                    certainly does not guide therapy. Treatment should
                    not be implemented on an out-patient basis as
                    parenteral antibiotics are required.

C R Whitfield in Ref 4

2.34 A **False**   Pelvic inflammatory disease characteristically causes
      B **True**   lower abdominal pain, backache, deep dyspareunia,
      C **True**   infertility and menstrual irregularities — the latter
      D **False**   probably due to ovarian dysfunction as a result of
      E **False**   recurrent episodes of infection. The disease being
                    chronic and low grade is not associated with pyrexia
                    or leucocytosis.

C R Whitfield in Ref 4

2.35 A **True**   Transient stress incontinence is common in the later
      B **True**   stages of pregnancy and in parous women. A bladder
      C **True**   support operation may be successful but may be
      D **True**   preceded by urodynamic studies if the nature of the
      E **True**   incontinence is not clear. Urodynamic studies have
                    shown low urethral closure pressure profiles in such
                    patients. Stress incontinence may occur without any
                    sign of prolapse.

L Cardozo in Ref 3 Vol 1

2.36 Urge incotinence in the female
A is worse during the day than at night
B may be due to a urinary tract infection
C is improved greatly by an anterior repair procedure
D is improved by bladder drill and re-education
E results in the daily passage of larger volumes or urine than normal

2.37 Urodynamic studies
A in upper motor neuronal diseases (e.g. multiple sclerosis) show an increased bladder capacity
B in stress incontinence reveal a detrusor pressure of between 20–30 cm of water
C should be performed in patients with apparently simple stress incontinence without urgency before considering therapy
D indicate the degree of elevation required for a curative colposuspension
E in the form of subtracted cystometry pressure will reveal detrusor instability

2.38 The following statements about a poor post-coital test are true:
A it is caused by sulphasalazine
B it is corrected by androgens
C it occurs in couples where the male has pus cells in the seminal fluid
D it is improved by 'condom therapy'
E serum anti-sperm antibodies can usually be demonstrated in the husband or wife if all the sperms are immotile or dead.

2.39 A dilatation and curettage
A is a useful treatment for dysmenorrhoea
B should be performed annually on postmenopausal patients taking oestrogens and progestogens
C is useful in the diagnosis of endometriosis
D aids the diagnosis of pelvic tuberculosis
E is useful in the diagnosis of a defective luteal phase

(*Answers overleaf*)

2.36 A **True**   The psychological element of this condition means
     B **True**   that sleep improves matters. However an insomniac
     C **False**   will remain the same! Urinary tract infection must be
     D **True**   excluded as a cause of any incontinence. Surgical
     E **False**   procedures are to be avoided in such situations as
                     there will be no improvement. An attempt to rectify
                     faulty attitude and bladder habit by bladder drill may
                     be successful. Although the patient micturates
                     frequently the daily urine output is unaffected.

L Cardozo in Ref 3 Vol 1

2.37 A **False**   Urodynamic studies should be performed in patients
     B **False**   with a complicated history of urinary incontinence
     C **False**   and in all those who have had previous surgery.
     D **False**   Detrusor instability shows on increased detrusor
     E **True**   pressure rise (above 15 cm of water) a day during
                     bladder filling or provocation testing. The usual
                     abnormality in MS is detrusor instability with
                     decreased bladder capacity. Genuine stress
                     incontinence shows no abnormality in simple
                     subtracted cystometry and the bladder neck
                     weakness is seen on radiographic screening.

L Cardozo in Ref 3 Vol 1

2.38 A **True**   A post coital test is an excellent screening test but the
     B **False**   interpretation of a negative or poor test is dificult. It
     C **True**   may occur when the male partner is taking drugs
     D **False**   such as sulphasalazine for inflammatory bowel
     E **False**   disease. It may occur in the presence of plasma or
                     mucous membrane antibodies, chronic seminal fluid
                     infection or simply because the test was not
                     performed at mid cycle. Treatment by condom
                     therapy, corticosteroids or artificial insemination by
                     husband is disappointing.

J Pryor in Ref 3 Vol 3

2.39 A **True**   Although by no means first-line therapy dilatation
     B **False**   and curettage frequently eases the pain of primary
     C **False**   dysmenorrhoea. It can be used to diagnose
     D **True**   endometrial tuberculosis but cannot help in the
     E **False**   diagnosis of endometriosis or defective luteal phase.
                     It is a much overused investigation in menstrual
                     disorders and can usually be performed as an
                     out-patient or suction curettage. This means of
                     endometrial sampling is useful as an annual screen
                     in postmenopausal patients taking unopposed
                     oestrogens without progestogens.

2.40 Gynaecological laparoscopy in the United Kingdom
A   is performed most commonly using carbon dioxide
B   carries a mortality of 8/100 000 cases
C   is associated with cardiac arrythmias
D   is associated with gas embolism
E   is suitable for post partum sterilization

2.41 Sterilization by the Pomeroy method
A   is performed with unabsorbable material
B   includes crushing the Fallopian tube
C   results in two separate ends of Fallopian tubes several
     months later
D   has a failure rate of about 0.3%
E   has a higher failure rate if performed at the time of Caesarean
     section

2.42 Unopposed oestrogen therapy for the post menopausal woman
A   improves the urethral syndrome
B   decreases urinary calcium excretion
C   causes decreased incidence of myocardial infarction
D   causes increased incidence of endometrial carcinoma
E   cause hypertension

2.43 Cryocautery to the cervix
A   requires freezing the cervix for 2 minutes
B   is performed with an IUCD in situ
C   requires para-cervical anaesthesia
D   leads to cervical dystocia
E   is effective treatment for CIN 3

(Answers overleaf)

2.40 A **True**   An RCOG working party made a Confidential Enquiry
     B **True**   into gynaecological laparoscopy reporting in 1978.
     C **True**   The most commonly used gas is carbon dioxide
     D **True**   although nitrous oxide is used in a few cases. The
     E **False**   mortality rate is 8/100 000 due to gas embolism,
                     cardiac arrest and anaesthetic complications.
                     Laparoscopy has a safety comparable with other
                     minor procedures but the complication rate of
                     laparoscopic sterilization was greater than diagnostic
                     laparoscopy. Anaesthetic problems should be
                     obviated by intubation.

Ref 23

2.41 A **False**   Sterilization must be performed using absorbable
     B **False**   suture material such as catgut and without crushing,
     C **True**   or a tubal fistula may occur between the two cut
     D **True**   ends. A portion of each tube is excised and once the
     E **True**   catgut has been absorbed the cut ends remain apart.
                     It has a failure rate of about one in three hundred and
                     this is much higher if it is performed at the time of
                     Caesarean section.

Ref 6

2.42 A **True**   Oestrogen therapy almost invariably removes the
     B **True**   classical climacteric symptoms of flushes, sweats
     C **False**   and atrophic vaginitis, as well as atrophic trigonitis
     D **True**   and the urethral syndrome. It decreases skeletal loss
     E **False**   and any excretion of calcium. It apparently has no
                     effect on the incidence of coronary thrombosis and it
                     must be accepted that unopposed oestrogen
                     increases the incidence of endometrial carcinoma.

D A Davey in Ref 4.

2.43 A **True**   Cryocautery to the cervix is a convenient cheap and
     B **True**   painless outpatient procedure. The freezing through
     C **False**   no more than 4 mm is inadequate for
     D **False**   carcinoma-in-situ. Cryocautery does not cause
     E **False**   cervical scarring.

J A Jordan in Ref 3 Vol 2

2.44 The following statements about cervical cytology are correct:
- **A** mass population screening programmes have not yet demonstrated a decrease in mortality from cervical carcinoma
- **B** dyskaryotic cells frequently convert to normal
- **C** malignant cells are characterised by a decreased nuclear/cytoplasmic ratio
- **D** grade II smears indicate the presence of infection
- **E** grade 5 smears indicate certain malignancy

2.45 The following features are visible in a fresh saline preparation of a vaginal discharge examined under the microscope:
- **A** desquamated epithelial cells
- **B** neisseria gonorrhoea
- **C** trichomonas vaginalis
- **D** candida albicans mycelia
- **E** spermatozoa

2.46 The contact hysteroscope
- **A** reveals a panoramic view of the uterine cavity
- **B** requires a viscous transluscent fluid for refraction
- **C** is used to identify vaginal foreign bodies
- **D** is used to diagnose pregnancy
- **E** uses ambient light

2.47 The following statements concerning uterine causes for are correct:
- **A** metroplasty, such as Strassman's operation, will improve the shape of the uterine cavity
- **B** a Foley's catheter is used to treat Asherman's syndrome
- **C** anti-tuberculous therapy may frequently restore fertility in endometrial tuberculosis
- **D** elective Caesarean section is indicated in a patient who has had a myomectomy
- **E** infertility due to uterine hypoplasia is helped by oestrogen therapy

(*Answers overleaf*)

2.44 A **False**   After ten years the Vancouver study has clearly
    B **True**   shown the benefits of population screening with a
    C **False**   decreased incidence and mortality of cervical
    D **True**   carcinoma. Superficial dyskaryotic cells (Grade 3)
    E **False**   may convert to normal, and Grade 5 malignant cells
still have to be investigated by biopsy, as the cervical
lesion may not be invasive. Malignant cells are
characterized by increased nuclear/cytoplasmic ratio,
irregular nuclear border and polychromatic staining
of the nucleus.

I D Duncan in Ref 3 Vol 1

2.45 A **True**   A fresh unstained preparation of vaginal discharge
    B **False**   will mostly show desquamated epithelial cells and
    C **True**   white cells although the motile Trichomonas
    D **False**   vaginalis and possibly spermatozoa may be seen.
    E **True**   Neisseria gonorrhoea requires gram staining to see
the intracellular diplococci and Candida albicans
mycelia also requires staining to be visible.

Ref 20

2.46 A **False**   The contact hysteroscope uses ambient light and
    B **False**   does not require any intra-uterine fluid. The angle of
    C **True**   vision is not panoramic but very limited. This
    D **True**   technique can be used to diagnose endometrial
    E **True**   polyps, identify the site of carcinoma, and even to
diagnose an early intra-uterine pregnancy without
disturbing it — hence an ectopic can be excluded. It is
most useful on occasions when a vaginal foreign
body is being sought in young children.

2.47 A **True**   Strassman's operation and myomectomy are
    B **True**   performed on the non gravid uterus and therefore the
    C **False**   risk of scar dehiscence in subsequent labour is
    D **False**   minimal. Uterine hypoplasia is a result of gonadal
    E **False**   insufficiency and oestrogen therapy will not improve
fertility. The infertility of pelvic tuberculosis is very
rarely corrected because of the gross tubal damage.

2.48 A vesico-vaginal fistula
  A   is associated with amenorrhoea
  B   is repaired by Franks technique
  C   is most commonly a result of obstructed labour in the United
      Kingdom
  D   should be left for ten days before repair
  E   is associated with pyelonephritis

2.49 The following surgical comments are true:
  A   urinary catheterization is necessary before vaginal
      hysterectomy
  B   six weeks should elapse between a cone biopsy and a
      Wertheim's hysterectomy
  C   Bonney's myomectomy clamps reduce post operative
      complications following myomectomy
  D   entry of the uterine cavity should be avoided at myomectomy
  E   the vaginal vault must be closed at an abdominal
      hysterectomy

2.50 A general micro-surgical principle is
  A   the use of a small skin incision
  B   irrigation of the operative field with water at body
      temperature
  C   the use of fine nylon sutures
  D   closure of all raw peritoneal areas
  E   magnification of x 25

(*Answers overleaf*)

2.48 A **True**   The incontinence due to a vesico-vaginal fistula
     B **False**   typically leads to constant wetness. In the developing
     C **False**   world most fistulae are due to obstructed labour but
     D **False**   in the United Kingdom most are subsequent to
     E **False**   gynaecological surgery or malignant disease of the
                   genital tract. A Martius graft of labial fat and fibrous
                   tissue facilitates repair. The Franks technique is a
                   non-surgical treatment for absence of the vagina.
                   Surprisingly ascending urinary tract infection is
                   uncommon probably because of constant flow and
                   absence of stasis. Coexistent amenorrhoea is very
                   common, presumably due to stress.

J Kelly in Ref 3 Vol 3

2.49 A **False**   Answers to surgical questions must be controversial
     B **False**   because surgical techniques are passed on from
     C **False**   teacher to pupil with the confidence and routine that
     D **False**   often defies scrutiny. It is our belief that it is
     E **False**   unnecessary and indeed wrong to empty the bladder
                   before vaginal hysterectomy. Similarly, Bonney's
                   clamps in our view increase the complications of
                   myomectomy by producing ischaemia and poor
                   intra-operative haemostasis. Cutting diathermy is
                   much to be preferred. Entry of the uterine cavity is
                   indicated in more extensive myomectomies in order
                   to observe the cavity and most importantly to
                   encourage drainage through the uterus rather than a
                   collection of pelvic blood clot. Vaginal vault closure is
                   optional. The patient with cervical cancer should not
                   wait six weeks before treatment.

2.50 A **False**   Microsurgery often means a macro-incision to enable
     B **False**   good exposure and minimal handling of tissue.
     C **True**   Ringer lactate solution (not water) at 40 °C should be
     D **True**   used as this prevents dessication and also facilitates
     E **True**   removal of blood from the peritoneal cavity. Nylon
                   rather than absorbable (i.e. rotting!) catgut or
                   polyglycolic acid sutures should be employed for
                   tubal surgery including all raw peritoneal surfaces.

R M L Winston in Ref 3 Vol 1

2.51 Tubal micro-surgery
A yields better results for ampullo-ampullary anastomosis than isthmo-isthmic anastomosis
B has a lower pregnancy rate if the tubes are short
C is facilitated by the use of indwelling prosthetic devices
D results in fewer ectopic pregnancies than following tubal macro-surgical techniques for similar lesions
E in the form of a salpingostomy in expert hands yields approximately a 30% intrauterine pregnancy rate

2.52 Black patients have a relatively increased incidence of
A fibroids
B endometriosis
C ectopic pregnancy
D rhesus disease
E diverticular disease

2.53 The following statements about genital prolapse are correct:
A recurrence is unusual following Le Fort's operation
B vaginal hysterectomy and pelvic floor repair is more effective than Manchester repair
C grade 4 uterine prolapse is a procidentia
D a Manchester repair includes cervical amputation and plication of the transverse cervical ligaments
E a ring pessary should be changed yearly

2.54 The following conditions should be treated by out-patient procedures:
A post-menopausal bleeding
B menorrhagia
C CIN 3
D 'pill' erosions
E Bartholin's cyst

(*Answers overleaf*)

2.51 A **False**   Best results are obtained if the tubes are long and if
     B **True**   an isthmo-isthmic anastomosis is performed but a
     C **False**   greater success in intrauterine pregnancy following
     D **False**   microsurgery usually means that there will be a
     E **False**   greater risk of ectopic pregnancy. The results of
                     salpingostomies are very poor — at the most 15% —
                     because the endosalpinges are invariably badly
                     damaged. Indwelling tubal prosthesis should not be
                     used as they destroy the function of the tubal
                     epithelium.

R M L Winston in Ref 3

2.52 A **True**   Black patients have a different incidence of certain
     B **False**   diseases which alters if environmental factors are
     C **True**   important when they adopt an urbanized life-style or
     D **False**   emigrate. They certainly have an increased incidence
     E **False**   of fibroids or ectopic pregnancy whilst endometriosis
                     and rhesus negative blood group are relatively rare.
                     Bowel disease is also less common on account of the
                     high roughage diet and that seems to apply
                     particularly to diverticular disease and appendicitis.

S Tuck in Ref 3 Vol 3

2.53 A **False**   Although the Manchester (Fothergill) procedure is a
     B **True**   useful and commonly performed operation, vaginal
     C **False**   hysterectomy is more likely to lead to cure and
     D **True**   removes the possibility of future menstrual problems
     E **False**   or uterine pathology. Recurrence after Le Fort's
                     operation is common and a vaginal hysterectomy
                     entails no greater morbidity. A ring pessary can be
                     used in these older patients but vaginal oestrogen
                     cream should be used and the pessary changed
                     every 4–6 months.

2.54 A **False**   Out-patient procedures in gynaecology are cost
     B **True**   effective and convenient for the patient. There are of
     C **True**   course limitations to their usefulness. Outpatient
     D **False**   suction currettage is excellent for the diagnosis of
     E **False**   menorrhagia but not post-menopausal bleeding
                     where there is a tight atrophic cervix and the
                     suspicion of malignancy is high. A Bartholin's cyst
                     requires a definitive procedure under anaesthesia. A
                     'pill' erosion should be treated by discontinuing or
                     changing the preparation and cervical intra-epithelial
                     type 3 lesion can be treated by out patient local
                     ablation.

2.55 Mastalgia is
- A associated with the polycystic ovarian syndrome
- B associated with an increased incidence of breast cancer
- C effectively treated with Danazol
- D often improved by combined oral contraceptive treatment
- E a part of the premenstrual syndrome

2.56 Cystic hyperplasia of the endometrium
- A is associated with herpes hominis type 2 infection
- B shows sub nuclear vacuolation in at least 50% of epithelial cells
- C produces polypoidal curettings
- D contains many stromal mitoses
- E is caused by unopposed oestrogen stimulation

2.57 Cystic hyperplasia
- A predisposes to carcinoma
- B does not occur in the post-menopause in the absence of oestrogen therapy
- C should be treated by the combined oral contraceptive in the perimenopausal woman
- D is treated with medroxyprogesterone acetate in preference to norethisterone
- E is associated with ovarian cysts

2.58 Congenital uterine abnormalities are associated with
- A hypotonic uterine action
- B ectopic pregnancy
- C post partum haemorrhage
- D dystocia
- E occipito-posterior position

(Answers overleaf)

2.55 A **False**   Mastalgia is a common and often ignored discomfort
B **True**   which is associated with abnormal duct patterns on
C **True**   mammography, so-called breast carcinoma-in-situ
D **True**   and a higher incidence of breast malignancy. It is
E **True**   associated with the pre-menstrual syndrome and in
general is probably caused by excess oestrogen
stimulation or the effect of progesterone following
ovulation. It is effectively treated with Danazol,
improved with the contraceptive pill and resolves
after the menopause.

2.56 A **False**   Cystic hyperplasia is now regarded as a better term
B **False**   than cystic glandular hyperplasia. It is an almost
C **True**   inevitable response to prolonged unopposed
D **True**   oestrogen therapy, produces thick polypoidal
E **True**   curettings and histologically is characterized by
hyperplasia of epithelial and stromal elements with
abundant mitotic figures. There is rarely subnuclear
vacuolation which would demonstrate a
progesterone effect.

Ref 20

2.57 A **False**   Cystic hyperplasia is associated with ovarian
B **False**   follicular cysts and anovulatory cycles. If a
C **False**   post-menopausal woman has a source of
D **True**   endogenous oestrogens hyperplasia can occur. It
E **True**   probably occurs in about 3% of woman after the
menopause. Carcinoma occurs in less than 0.3% of
patients with cystic hyperplasia and the consensus is
that it is not a pre-malignant condition. It is best
treated by progestagen and current evidence shows
that medroxyprogesterone does not have the
adverse effect on lipids found with other
progestagens.

Ref 20

2.58 A **False**   Early pregnancy wastage is associated with the
B **True**   various degrees of uterine malfusion. Ectopic
C **True**   pregnancy occurs in a rudimentary horn. Later
D **True**   pregnancy may be complicated by abnormal lie,
E **False**   premature labour, abormal labour, retained placenta
and post partum haemorrhage. Abnormal labour is
more likely to be due to abnormal lie than abnormal
position or abnormal uterine action.

Ref 6

2.59 The following statements about eponymous operations are appropriate:
A   McIndoe-Read and vaginoplasty
B   Moscovitz and enterocoele
C   Fothergill and vaginal hysterectomy
D   Burch and anterior repair
E   Schauta and carcinoma of the cervix

2.60 Which of the following associations are correct:
A   Meig's syndrome and fibroids
B   Krukenberg tumours and carcinoma of the colon
C   Martius graft and stress incontinence
D   Lawson Tait and ovariotomy
E   Marion Sims and slaves

2.61 High gonadotrophin levels are found in
A   ovarian teratoma
B   Sheehan's syndrome
C   mosaicism with a Y chromosome
D   climacteric patients with regular cycles
E   17 hydroxylase deficiency

2.62 Mycoplasma
A   causes male infertility
B   is Gram-negative
C   can be successfully treated with penicillin
D   causes neonatal pneumonia
E   causes pelvic inflammatory disease

2.63 Mycoplasma
A   is a virus
B   causes Reiter's syndrome
C   causes low birth weight babies
D   causes salpingitis
E   causes acute pyelonephritis

(Answers overleaf)

2.59 A **True**   The McIndoe-Read is a classical operation for absent
     B **True**   vagina which includes skin grafting. This has been
     C **False**   superceded by the Williams operation, which creates
     D **False**   a pouch from the asexual skin of the perineum. The
     E **True**   Moscovitz operation is an abdominal approach to an
                     enterocoele and the Burch operation is a
                     colposuspension for genuine stress incontinence.
                     The Fothergill operation is synonymous with
                     Manchester repair and a Schauta is a radical vaginal
                     hysterectomy with iliac node dissection.

Ref D Lees & A Singer in Ref 24

2.60 A **False**   Lawson Tait and Marion Sims were great pioneers of
     B **True**   gynaecology. Lawson Tait was famous for removing
     C **False**   ovarian tumours and Marion Sims for repairing
     D **True**   vesico-vaginal fistulae initially in slaves. The Martius
     E **True**   graft is the creation of a pedicle from the labia with
                     adequate blood supply facilitating repair of a
                     vesico-vaginal fistulae.

2.61 A **True**   Elevated gonadotrophin levels occur in peri
     B **False**   menopausal women before the cessation of menses,
     C **True**   Turner's syndrome, premature ovarian failure and
     D **True**   most abnormal karyotypes when there is a Y
     E **True**   chromosome present. It is important to recognise the
                     importance of a Y chromosome as this patient may
                     require laparotomy and gonadectomy. Malignant
                     tumours such as ovarian teratoma frequently have a
                     raised FSH.

Ref 12

2.62 A **True**   Mycoplasma is a Gram-negative organism with both
     B **True**   viral and bacterial characteristics. It is a sexually
     C **False**   transmitted disease causing chronic epididymitis,
     D **True**   salpingitis and neonatal jaundice. Treatment is by
     E **True**   tetracycline or ampicillin.

M J Emens in Ref 3 Vol 3

2.63 A **False**   Mycoplasma is neither a virus nor a bacterium but
     B **False**   has some properties characteristic of each. It is
     C **True**   becoming apparent that both Mycoplasma and
     D **True**   Chlamydia are common causes of non-specific
     E **True**   urethritis and salpingitis. Mycoplasma also causes
                     acute pyelonephritis and, reasons unknown, low
                     birth weight babies.

M J Emens in Ref 3 Vol 3

2.64 Anaerobic infections
A   are usually poly-microbic
B   are usually from exogenous sources
C   by bacteroides usually have an accompanying bacteraemia
D   are effectively treated by chloramphenicol
E   if treated by clindamycin may be complicated by a peripheral neuropathy

2.65 Childhood vulvovaginitis
A   is commonly due to staphylococcal infection
B   is commonly due to Monilia
C   is caused by threadworm infestation
D   is treated with oestrogen cream
E   commonly requires treatment with systemic antibiotics

2.66 Congenital absence of the vagina is associated with
A   absent secondary sexual characteristics
B   absent uterus
C   exposure to diethyl stilboestrol in utero
D   Turner's syndrome
E   imperforate anus

2.67 Uterus didelphys is associated with
A   oligomenorrhoea
B   transverse lie of the fetus
C   urinary tract abnormalities
D   failure of fusion of mesonephric ducts
E   Downs syndrome

(*Answers overleaf*)

2.64 A **True**   Anaerobic infections are almost invariably mixed and
      B **False**   come from endogenous sources. They are difficult to
      C **True**   culture but bacteroides infections often have
      D **True**   co-existent septicaemia and may be recognized by
      E **False**   blood culture. Clindamycin may cause fatal
                    necrotising enteritis and although chloramphenicol
                    may rarely in large doses produce aplastic anaemia,
                    it is a very effective treatment, is cheap and has a
                    certain place in developing countries where the
                    newer antibiotics are either very expensive or not
                    available.

I Brown in Ref 3 Vol 2

2.65 A **False**   Vulvovaginitis in chidhood is usually due to a mixed
      B **False**   growth of organisms of low pathogenicity.
      C **True**   Threadworm infestation is a recognized cause and
      D **True**   requires specific treatment. A foreign body causes
      E **False**   foul discharge which may be bloodstained, and if this
                    is the case rectal examination or examination under
                    anaesthesia should be performed. Non-specific
                    treatment, attention to hygiene and clothing is
                    usually adequate, but oestrogen cream provides
                    relief by increasing natural protection. Systemic
                    antibiotic are unnecessary unless a specific pathogen
                    is recognized.

C J Dewhurst in Ref 4

2.66 A **False**   Most cases of absent vagina also have an absent
      B **True**   uterus but ovaries are present because of their
      C **False**   different embryological origin. Secondary sexual
      D **False**   characteristics therefore appear normally. Turner's
      E **False**   syndrome includes abnormal ovaries and a small
                    uterus.

Ref 12

2.67 A **False**   Duplication of the uterus and cervix may have no
      B **False**   clinical manifestation although menorrhagia due to
      C **True**   increased area of endometrium and obstructive
      D **False**   labour due to the non-pregnant half are recorded. It is
      E **False**   the paramesonephric (Mullerian) ducts which fail to
                    fuse and any genital tract abnormality may be
                    associated with urinary tract abnormalities.

C J Dewhurst in Ref 4

2.68 The Wolffian duct is the origin of
  A   Walthard's rests
  B   Gartner's duct
  C   parovarian cysts
  D   gynandroblastoma
  E   streak gonads in XY gonadal dysgenesis

2.69 Vaginal septa are associated with
  A   dyspareunia
  B   dysmenorrhoea
  C   obstructed labour
  D   uterine abnormalities
  E   exposure to stilboestrol in utero

2.70 The following plasma hormones peak at the middle of a normal menstrual cycle:
  A   testosterone
  B   follicle stimulating hormone
  C   17 alpha hydroxy progesterone
  D   oestradiol
  E   adrenocorticotrophic hormone

2.71 In the normal ovary
  A   primordial follicles arise from the germinal epithelium
  B   the theca externa is a false capsule of connective tissue
  C   the corpus luteum is formed from theca cells
  D   the primary oocyte is haploid
  E   oogenesis continues until puberty

2.72 The following features are characteristic of cervical mucus in mid cycle:
  A   increased quantity
  B   increased cellularity
  C   absence of arborization
  D   increased viscosity
  E   the presence of red cells

(Answers overleaf)

2.68 A **False**   Wolffian duct development, although suppressed in
    B **True**   the female, may leave residual structures parallel to
    C **True**   the developed Mullerian ducts which form the genital
    D **False**   tract. Para vaginal cysts and parovarian cysts occur.
    E **False**   Walthard's rests are squamous metaplasia found
        within the cortex of the ovary. Gynandroblastoma
        and streak gonads develop from the primitive genital
        ridge.

Ref 12

2.69 A **True**   Vaginal septa in the sagittal plane are associated with
    B **False**   uterine and urinary tract anomalies. Dyspareunia
    C **True**   occurs and labour may be obstructed especially in
    D **True**   breech presentation. Stilboestrol has no association
    E **False**   with this condition.

C J Dewhurst in Ref 4

2.70 A **False**   FSH, LH and serum oestrogens peak in mid-cycle
    B **True**   coincident with ovulation. Progesterone and 17-alpha
    C **False**   hydroxy progesterone peak in the luteal phase of
    D **True**   the cycle. ACTH adrenal hormones and testosterone
    E **False**   do not rise to a peak related to the menstrual cycle.

Ref 4

2.71 A **False**   The primordial follicles and germ cells develop
    B **True**   within the ovarian substance not from the
    C **False**   inappropriately named germinal epithelium which
    D **False**   surrounds the ovary. Oogenesis ceases during intra-
    E **False**   uterine life and from then on most oocytes become
        atretic. The first reduction division converts the
        diploid primary oocyte into the haploid secondary
        oocyte. The corpus luteum forms from granulosa
        cells.

M C MacNaughton in Ref 5

2.72 A **True**   Cervical mucus in mid cycle is affected by oestrogen
    B **False**   stimulation. It is increased in amount, clear and thin.
    C **False**   It exhibits spinnbarkeit being less viscous and when
    D **False**   dried on a microscope slide shows arborization
    E **False**   (ferning) but red cells are not seen. It is usefully
        assessed at mid cycle in the post coital test when
        surviving sperm migration is also assessed.

C J Dewhurst in Ref 4

2.73 In normal puberty the following features are characteristic:
A pubic hair growth is the first sign
B axillary hair growth occurs after the first menstrual period
C the first menstrual cycles are anovulatory
D cessation of growth
E changes in the vaginal epithelium

2.74 Precocious puberty in the female is associated with
A testicular feminization
B encephalitis
C arrhenoblastoma
D olfacto-genital syndrome
E Albrights syndrome

2.75 The Barr body
A occurs in 90% of cells in the female
B occurs in 20% of cells in the male
C appears as a dense rod close to the cell wall
D occurs in Klinefelters syndrome
E is always derived from paternal X chromosomes

2.76 Patients with testicular feminization characteristically
A are XY mosaic
B have a hypoplastic uterus
C are chromatin positive
D have poorly developed breasts
E have pure gonadal dysgenesis

2.77 Characteristic features of Klinefelters syndrome include
A mental retardation
B oligospermia
C gynaecomastia
D XYY genotype
E congenital heart disease

(*Answers overleaf*)

2.73 A **False**   Normal puberty commences with breast
     B **False**   development and the start of a growth spurt which
     C **True**   continues throughout. It is followed by pubic hair
     D **False**   development, axillary hair and then the first
     E **True**   menstrual period (the menarche). Changes occur in
                    the vaginal epithelium due to oestrogen stimulation.

C J Dewhurst in Ref 4

2.74 A **False**   Precocious puberty in the female is usually
     B **True**   constitutional but intracranial lesions and feminizing
     C **False**   ovarian tumours must be excluded. Olfacto-genital
     D **False**   syndrome (Kallmann's syndrome in its familial form)
     E **True**   and testicular feminization are both associated with
                    amenorrhoea. In Albrights syndrome polyostotic
                    fibrous dysplasia and cafe au lait spots on the skin are
                    associated with precocious puberty.

C J Dewhurst in Ref 4

2.75 A **False**   The Barr body, named after its discoverer, represents
     B **False**   one of the X chromosomes, lies close to the nuclear
     C **False**   membrane and may be of maternal or paternal
     D **True**   origin. It occurs in about 50% of cells in normal
     E **False**   females and does not occur in males, and is
                    numerically one less than the number of X
                    chromosomes. Klinefelters syndrome (XXY) although
                    phenotypically a male, has one Barr body.

J S Scott in Ref 14

2.76 A **False**   Amenorrhoeic women of genotype XY may have
     B **False**   testicular feminization or pure gonadal dysgenesis.
     C **False**   Having one X chromosome they are chromatin
     D **False**   negative. Patients with testicular feminization have a
     E **False**   blind vagina, no uterus, but well-developed breasts.
                    Gonadal dysgenesis is associated with streak gonads
                    and a hypoplastic uterus.

J S Scott in Ref 14

2.77 A **False**   Klinefelters syndrome occurs in phenotypic males
     B **False**   with XXY genotype. Azoospermia is the rule and
     C **True**   infertility a feature. Gynaecomastia and
     D **False**   eunuchoidism occur but congenital heart disease is
     E **False**   not a feature. While patients with Klinefelters
                    syndrome are more often mentally retarded than
                    other males, it is not a characteristic feature.

J S Scott in Ref 14

2.78 In true hermaphroditism
A external sex is usually female
B chromosomal sex is usually female (46XX)
C mosaics do not occur
D primordial follicles and seminiferous tubules are both present
E end-organ resistance is a feature

2.79 Patients with testicular feminization
A have streak gonads
B have high testosterone levels
C have high gonadotrophin levels
D need removal of gonads before puberty
E are often hirsute

2.80 Primary amenorrhoea is associated with
A craniopharyngioma
B testicular feminization
C congenital adrenal hyperplasia
D coeliac disease
E virilizing male intersex

2.81 Sexual infantilism is consistent with a diagnosis of
A congenital adrenal hyperplasia
B Laurence-Moon-Biedl syndrome
C ateliotic dwarfism
D true gonadal agenesis
E Kallmann's syndrome

2.82 The following features are associated with secondary amenorrhoea:
A thyrotoxicosis
B bicornate uterus
C Asherman's syndrome
D pelvic tuberculosis
E virilizing ovarian tumour

(*Answers overleaf*)

2.78 A **False**   In this condition both primordial follicles and
      B **True**   seminiferous tubules are present in gonadal tissue.
      C **False**   Chromosomal structure is usually 46XX. Mosaics do
      D **True**   occur but external sex is predominantly male with a
      E **False**   phallus while a uterus is commonly present.

R P Shearman in Ref 4

2.79 A **False**   Testicular feminization patients have high
      B **True**   gonadotrophin and testosterone levels. They have
      C **True**   testes in the inguinal canal as a hernia or in the labia.
      D **False**   As there is increased incidence of gonadal
      E **False**   malignancy (dysgerminoma) they should be
                     removed after puberty as the testes are necessary for
                     normal development. Typically these patients have
                     scanty body and sexual hair.

J S Scott in Ref 14

2.80 A **True**   Primary amenorrhoea is caused by disorders of the
      B **True**   hypo-thalamo-pituitary-ovarian axis and anatomical
      C **True**   abnormalities of the genital organs. Chromosomal
      D **True**   abnormalities and intersex states of which there is a
      E **True**   complex classification are also associated. General
                     systemic diseases leading to stunting of growth and
                     immaturity are also causes. Late onset adrenal
                     hyperplasia and virilizing disorders also cause this.

R P Shearman in Ref 4

2.81 A **False**   Sexual infantilism implies the absence of any sex
      B **True**   hormone secretion. It occurs in Turner's syndrome
      C **True**   and true gonadal agenesis due to ovarian failure of
      D **True**   development. It also occurs in ateliotic dwarfism due
      E **True**   to pituitary failure, and in Laurence-Moon-Biedl
                     syndrome due to congenital hypothalamo-pituitary
                     disturbance.

R P Shearman in Ref 4

2.82 A **True**   Any systemic illness may be associated with
      B **False**   secondary amenorrhoea but especially psychiatric
      C **True**   disorders, uncontrolled diabetes mellitus,
      D **True**   thyrotoxicosis and tuberculosis. Tuberculosis of the
      E **True**   endometrium and amenorrhoea traumatica
                     (Asherman's syndrome) cause amenorrhoea by local
                     effects.

R D Shearman in Ref 4

2.83 Patients with pure gonadal dysgenesis
A   are usually XO or mosaic
B   always have primary amenorrhoea
C   have a uterus
D   have neck webbing
E   have normal breasts

2.84 Asherman's syndrome
A   is characterized by infertility, recurrent abortion and menorrhagia
B   occurs after puerperal curettage
C   is associated with obstetric complications including post partum haemorrhage
D   may be treated by forceps
E   may be treated by a Foley catheter

2.85 Cervical imcompetence
A   is a common cause of first trimester abortion
B   may be congenital
C   is associated with previous instrumental delivery
D   is diagnozed by follicular phase hysterography
E   is associated with painless premature labour

2.86 The following features suggest a diagnosis of ectopic pregnancy:
A   amenorrhoea of fourteen weeks
B   Arias stella reaction on endometrial histology
C   normal sized uterus
D   heavy vaginal bleeding
E   decidual tissue at curettage

(Answers overleaf)

2.83 A **False**   Patients with pure gonadal dysgenesis are usually XY
     B **True**   or can be mosaic. They have streak gonads, primary
     C **True**   amenorrhoea but no stigmata of Turner's syndrome.
     D **False**   Unlike XY patients with testicular feminization they
     E **False**   have small immature breasts.

R P Shearman in Ref 4

2.84 A **False**   Asherman's syndrome produces infertility and
     B **True**   amenorrhoea and more frequently occurs following
     C **True**   puerperal curettage than after termination. Treatment
     D **False**   is difficult but encouraging results have been
     E **True**   obtained by priming the endometrium with
                    oestrogen and inserting an intracavity Foley catheter
                    or intrauterine device for two weeks. There is a high
                    incidence of subsequent difficult pregnancy
                    especially pathological adherence of the placenta and
                    therefore post partum haemorrhage.

Ref 12

2.85 A **False**   Cervical incompetence causes second trimester
     B **True**   abortion and characteristically a rapid and painless
     C **True**   premature delivery. Congenital cases are seen but
     D **False**   more commonly there is a history of interference
     E **True**   with the cervix, previous dilatation, cone biopsy or
                    instrumental delivery. Hysterography using a
                    Leech-Wilkinson cannula only confirms the diagnosis
                    in the premenstrual phase. It is believed by many that
                    the diagnosis cannot be made by hysterography but
                    it is a functional diagnosis obtained from the history.

J S Scott in Ref 4

2.86 A **False**   The period of amenorrhoea in ectopic pregnancy is
     B **True**   usually six to ten weeks. The uterus is normally
     C **False**   enlarged due to endocrine changes of pregnancy.
     D **False**   The endometrium shows decidual changes and the
     E **True**   glandular atypia of the Arias stella reaction may be
                    found in up to 20% of cases. Sporadic bleeding is
                    usually scanty with altered blood and comes from the
                    decidua not the damaged tube.

N Kadar in Ref 3 Vol 3

2.87 Ectopic pregnancy
A is commoner in the right fallopian tube
B is commoner in intrauterine device users than in patients using no contraception.
C is associated with pelvic tuberculosis
D is associated with tubal surgery for infertility
E is commonly ovarian

2.88 The following statements about ectopic pregnancy are true:
A the ipsi-lateral ovary should be removed
B a tender adnexal mass strongly suggests the diagnosis
C the afffected tube must be removed
D diagnostic laparoscopy should precede laparotomy
E more than half the deaths in the United Kingdom are in black patients

2.89 In the differentiation of ectopic gestation from acute pelvic inflammatory disease the following results of investigations would be helpful:
A a white cell count of 10 000/cu mm
B an erythrocyte sedimentation rate (ESR) of 35 mm/hour
C a laparoscopic finding of blood in the peritoneal cavity
D a negative pregnancy test
E negative culdocentesis for blood

(Answers overleaf)

2.87 A **True**   The most common aetiological factor in patients with
      B **False**   ectopic pregnancy is previous pelvic inflammation.
      C **True**   The incidence in different communities varies
      D **True**   greatly. Whilst ectopic pregnancies occur in patients
      E **False**   with intrauterine contraceptive devices, it is less
                       common than in the general population and
                       intrauterine contraceptive devices cannot be said to
                       cause the condition. Tubal abnormalities, infertility,
                       previous tubal surgery and previous appendicitis are
                       strong associations.

J S Scott in Ref 4

2.88 A **False**   Although still an area of debate it is generally
      B **False**   accepted that a functioning endocrine organ should
      C **False**   not be removed. Contrary to the statements of many
      D **False**   standard texts the finding of a tender adnexal mass
      E **True**   usually suggests that the pathology is not an ectopic.
                       There is often a good case for achieving haemostasis
                       if possible and leaving the affected tube. The
                       diagnosis and the need for laparotomy is often too
                       clear to waste time performing a laparoscopy. The
                       racial difference in mortality is an important area for
                       further study.

N Kadar in Ref 3 Vol 3

2.89 A **False**   This is a common clinical problem and the only
      B **False**   conclusive investigation in the presence of a clinical
      C **True**   suspicion of ectopic pregnancy is laparoscopy. The
      D **False**   white cell count and ESR may be raised in both
      E **False**   conditions although a very high white cell count
                       would suggest inflammation. A pregnancy test may
                       be negative in ectopic pregnancy if the trophoblast is
                       no longer viable and has ceased to produce human
                       chorionic gonadotrophin. A positive pregnancy test
                       would suggest ectopic pregnancy but there may then
                       be doubt if a pregnancy is intra uterine or extra
                       uterine. Culdocentesis may not produce blood even
                       although there is a haemoperitoneum.

N Kadar in Ref 3 Vol 3

2.90 Incarceration of the retroverted gravid uterus
A characteristically occurs about ten weeks' gestation
B presents commonly with stress incontinence
C is treated by bimanual manipulation
D causes difficulty in palpating the cervix on vaginal examination
E is treated by urethral catheterization

2.91 During normal sexual response
A vaginal lubrication occurs from cervical and vulval glands
B uterine size increases
C the 'orgasmic platform' of the upper third of the vagina occurs
D a 'sex flush' occurs around the perineum
E the resolution phase precedes the orgasm

2.92 The following statements about sexual dysfunction in young women are true:
A Hormone changes are associated with loss of libido
B The 'sensate focus' therapy involves prohibition of intercourse
C Testosterone therapy improves loss of libido
D Vaginismus is most commonly organic in aetiology
E Anorgasmia produces pelvic pathology

2.93 Spontaneous abortion
A occurs in at least 20% of pregnancies
B has been the most frequent cause of maternal death in England and Wales
C is often associated with fetal abnormality
D is associated with malaria
E is prevented by progestagen injection

(*Answers overleaf*)

2.90 A **False**   Incarceration of the retroverted gravid uterus
     B **False**   presents between twelve and sixteen weeks'
     C **False**   gestation with urinary retention. The cervix is drawn
     D **True**   upwards and may be inpalpable while the uterus
     E **True**   itself is felt as a palpable mass in the posterior
                   vaginal fornix. Manipulation is contra-indicated,
                   sometimes precipitating abortion. Urethral
                   catheterization and postural treatment effect a cure.

C J Dewhurst in Ref 4

2.91 A **False**   Vaginal lubrication occurs as a transudation through
     B **True**   the vagina from surrounding congestion. The uterus
     C **False**   increases in size, the upper third of the vagina
     D **False**   balloons and the thickened orgasmic platform occurs
     E **False**   in the lower third of the vagina. The sex flush is a
                   generalized skin hyperaemia. Resolution follows
                   orgasm.

T Betts in Ref 3 Vol 2

2.92 A **False**   Although no specific hormone changes can be found
     B **True**   with libido loss, therapy with Testosterone can
     C **True**   improve this condition. The 'sensate focus' involves
     D **False**   physical stimulation with the fear of intercourse
     E **True**   removed. Vaginismus is nearly always psychological
                   and sexual stimulation without orgasm can (and
                   probably commonly does) produce pelvic pathology
                   in the form of congestion and deep pelvic pain.

T Betts in Ref 3 Vol 2

2.93 A **True**   20% is considered a low figure and some authorities
     B **False**   suggest 30% would be correct. Between 1955 and
     C **True**   1972 abortion was the most common cause of death
     D **True**   but this included illegal induced abortion. Perhaps
     E **False**   50% of abortions have been shown to have
                   chromosomal abnormalities. Any infective or
                   metabolic upset may precipitate abortion. Controlled
                   studies have shown no improvement in the rate of
                   continuance of pregnancy in patients treated with
                   progestagens.

J S Scott in Ref 4

2.94 Termination of pregnancy
A is controlled in the United Kingdom by 1967 Abortion Act
B is safely performed per vaginam at eighteen weeks' gestation
C is performed using extra amniotic hypertonic saline
D carries a risk of sensitization in rhesus negative women
E carries a mortality in the first trimester of 5/100 000 cases

2.95 Oral contraception is associated with
A a pregnancy rate of about 1/1000 woman years
B increased risk of endometriosis
C crises in porphyric patients
D a mortality of 1.4/100 000 in young non-smoking women
E a mortality of 15/100 000 women over the age of 35 who smoke

2.96 Ultrasonography in early pregnancy
A can diagnose ectopic pregnancy
B can pick up the fetal heart at 8 weeks of amenorrhoea
C will demonstrate a crown-rump length of 30 mm at 8 weeks
D may confuse a hydatidiform mole with a fibroid
E can diagnose an intra-uterine gestational sac after 5 weeks of amenorrhoea

2.97 The following associations are appropriate:
A ascaris lumbricoides and menorrhagia
B ankylostoma duodenale and pruritis vulvae
C enterobius vermicularis and anaemia
D schistosoma haematobium and haematuria
E malaria and tubal damage

(*Answers overleaf*)

2.94 A **True**   The 1967 Abortion Act controls this type of procedure
     B **False**   in the UK but it may only be carried out with safety
     C **False**   per vaginam until twelve to fourteen weeks'
     D **True**   gestation. After that an infusion of extra amniotic
     E **False**   prostaglandin is one of the methods used to
precipitate abortion. Hypertonic saline has been used
intra amniotically but is not recommended. There is a
risk of rhesus sensitization and all such women
should have anti-D immunoglobulin within 48 hours.
Mortality is related to length of gestation and is about
4/100 000 in Britain. It may be half this in the early
first trimester and four times this in the second
trimester.

Ref 19

2.95 A **True**   There is a reduced risk of endometriesis, breast
     B **False**   cancer and endometrial cancer in women taking the
     C **True**   oral contraceptive. The mortality of 1.4/100 000 in
     D **True**   young, non-smoking women is increased to over
     E **False**   30/100 000 in women over the age of 35 and who
smoke.

Ref 19

2.96 A **True**   Ultrasound can often pick up an ectopic pregnancy in
     B **True**   a patient with a full bladder. Alternatively an intra
     C **False**   uterine pregnancy virtually excludes it. A
     D **True**   degenerating fibroid can be mis-diagnosed as a
     E **True**   hydatidiform mole as those of us who have tried to
induce labour in such a case will confirm.

S Campbell in Ref 3 Vol 3

2.97 A **False**   Infestations are not uncommon in patients from
     B **False**   Africa — if you look for them. An important cause of
     C **False**   anaemia is hookworm (ankylostoma) and malaria.
     D **True**   Bilharzia (schistosomiasis) causes haematuria.
     E **False**   Pruritis vulvae in children is caused by the more
ubiquitous threadworm (Enteribius vermicularis).

S Wood in Ref 5

2.98 Adenomyosis
    A has its origin in Mullerian rests in the myometrium
    B can undergo malignant change to adenocarcinoma
    C is associated with a high incidence of endometrial hyperplasia
    D is associated with a higher incidence of pelvic (external) endometriosis
    E is associated with a low grade sarcomatous change

2.99 Herpes-virus hominis (HVH)
    A type I invades the oral mucosa
    B type I does not involve the genital organs
    C type II may infect the baby at delivery in approximately 40% of cases
    D type II infection of the neonate usually manifests itself in the first and second days of life
    E type I has an aetiological role in carcinoma of the ovary

2.100 Chronic pelvic infection
    A is associated with utero-sacral thickening
    B yields positive peritoneal bacterial cultures in 50% of cases
    C has positive serology for gonorrhoea in 20% of cases
    D shows a good response to long term antibiotic therapy
    E usually requires removal of ovaries at the time of hysterectomy

2.101 The following are symptoms of the climacteric:
    A obesity
    B premenstrual tension
    C formication
    D menorrhagia
    E headaches

(*Answers overleaf*)

2.98 A **False**   Adenomyosis is not as previously thought due to
     B **True**   rests from Mullerian or Wolffian ducts, but is a
     C **True**   downgrowth of the endometrium of uterine cavity
     D **True**   associated with both endometrial hyperplasia and
     E **True**   endometriosis. Adenocarcinoma can occur within
                   one of the endometrial areas and this is an important
                   distinction when considering depth of invasion from
                   an apparent endometrial carcinoma. Stromal
                   endometriosis is a low grade malignancy of the
                   stroma.

E Novak & J D Woodruff in Ref 20

2.99 A **True**   Herpes virus type I infects the oral mucosa and type II
     B **False**   the genital tract, although there is much oro-genital
     C **True**   transmission of type I to the vulva. They are not
     D **False**   distinguishable by electron-microscopy and indeed
     E **False**   might be the same virus. 40% of babies are affected if
                   the lesion is active. The risk is less following delivery
                   by Caesarean section. The child appears normal at
                   birth, but a very severe systemic disease occurs in
                   the first month of life.

2.100 A **True**   The cause of chronic pelvic infection may be
      B **False**   pyogenic, gonococcal or tuberculous, but cultures
      C **False**   are very rarely helpful. Clinical findings include
      D **False**   tender retroversion and adnexal and uterosacral
      E **True**   thickening. Medical therapy is disappointing for long
                    term relief and hysterectomy without oophorectomy
                    often leads to recurrence of pain. It is usually best to
                    remove ovaries and give the patient long term
                    oestrogen therapy.

C R Whitfield in Ref 4

2.101 A **False**   The most characteristic features of the climacteric are
      B **False**   the vasomotor symptoms of hot flushes, sweats and
      C **True**   headaches. Menstrual disturbances are not regarded
      D **False**   as a normal feature of the approaching menopuase.
      E **True**   The itching under the skin known as formication is
                    unusual but characteristic.

R Greenblatt & J W W Studd in Ref 5

2.102 The following statements about premenstrual tension are correct:
  A   there is characteristically abnormal plasma hormone profiles
  B   there is characteristically an abnormal premorbid personality
  C   it is improved by progestagen therapy
  D   it is improved by combined oral contraceptive therapy
  E   it is associated with a past history of post-partum depression.

2.103 Lippes loop intra-uterine contraceptive devices
  A   no longer have a significant place in contraceptive practice
  B   need to be changed every five years
  C   are associated with pelvic actinomycosis
  D   are associated with Bechet's syndrome
  E   can be detected in the uterine cavity if 'lost' by straight A P pelvic X-ray

2.104 Inert intra-uterine contraceptive devices
  A   using monofilament nylon threads have been incriminated in causing fatal sepsis
  B   should be changed every two years
  C   pre-dispose to congenital limb deformities
  D   should not be used in patients with valvular heart disease
  E   act by creating a hostile uterine environment

2.105 The following metabolic changes occur after the menopause:
  A   decreased plasma testosterone
  B   decreased plasma calcium
  C   decreased plasma luteinizing hormone
  D   decreased plasma androstenedione
  E   decreased plasma cholesterol

2.106 Combined oestrogen/progestogen contraceptive pills
  A   were first used on a large scale in humans in 1946
  B   contain either ethinyl oestradiol or mestranol as the oestrogen component
  C   characteristically regularise and reduce vaginal bleeding
  D   should not be used in patients with liver disease
  E   are associated with an increased incidence of thrombo embolic episodes

(*Answers overleaf*)

2.102 A **False**   The clearest indictment of the understanding of
      B **True**   premenstrual tension is the lack of any facts about its
      C **False**   pathology or treatment. Perhaps it does not exist!
      D **True**   There have been no characteristic hormone changes
      E **True**   elucidated nor any effective therapy demonstrated by
                    double blind placebo trials. The syndrome is clearly
                    due to a change in various hormones following
                    ovulation and suppression of ovulation is usually
                    helpful, although the progestagenic component of
                    the pill may exacerbate symptoms.

A Magos in Ref 3 Vol 4

2.103 A **False**   Lippes loops still have a place because they do not
      B **False**   need changing. The infection rate is probably no
      C **True**   higher than a copper device although there is a
      D **False**   certain association with pelvic actinomycosis.
      E **False**   Detection and positioning by X-ray can only be
                    achieved by an antero-posterior plus lateral X-ray
                    with a probe in the uterine cavity.

Ref 19

2.104 A **False**   Intra-uterine contraceptive devices are thought to act
      B **False**   mainly by creating a hostile intra-uterine
      C **False**   environment. It is recommended that copper devices
      D **True**   should be changed every two years, but other
      E **True**   devices may remain in place for longer intervals.
                    They may provide a portal of entry for bacteria and
                    there is a risk of endocarditis in patients with valvular
                    heart disease, and also severe sepsis with the
                    braided nylon thread of the Dalkon shield.

Ref 19

2.105 A **False**   The endocrine changes after the menopause are a
      B **False**   decrease in oestrone, oestradiol and
      C **False**   androstenedione. There is elevation in
      D **True**   gonadotrophins and no change in plasma
      E **False**   testosterone. Plasma cholesterol and calcium increase.

R B Greenblatt & J W W Studd in Ref 5

2.106 A **False**   Oral contraceptives were first introduced in Puerto
      B **True**   Rico in 1956. They may contain either ethinyl
      C **True**   oestradiol or mestranol but the mestranol is
      D **True**   converted in the body to ethinyl oestradiol. Liver
      E **True**   disease and a history of thrombosis are important
                    contra-indications to their use.

Ref 19

2.107 **The following are features of altered lipid metabolism in women taking combined oral contraceptive preparations:**
A   decreased free fatty acids
B   increased triglycerides
C   decreased cholesterol
D   increased beta lipoprotein
E   oestrogen dose dependence

2.108 **Metabolic changes that occur on the combined oestrogen progestogen oral contraceptive are:**
A   increased triglycerides
B   decreased serum albumin
C   carbohydrate intolerance
D   increased serum anti Xa (anti-thrombin III)
E   decreased prolactin

2.109 **The unruptured luteinised follicle**
A   usually occurs with abnormal luteal plasma hormone levels
B   is associated with endometriosis
C   does not have a corpus luteum stigma
D   is associated with greater concentrations of 17-Beta oestradiol and progesterone in the peritoneal fluid
E   may be diagnozed by laparoscopy in the week after supposed ovulation.

2.110 **Progestogen therapy produces the following complications:**
A   Dowager's hump
B   mastalgia
C   acne
D   premenstrual tension
E   cholestasis

(*Answers overleaf*)

2107 A **False**   Triglycerides, free fatty acids, cholesterol and beta
     B **True**   lipoproteins are elevated in women taking combined
     C **False**   oral contraceptive pills. This is an oestrogen effect, is
     D **True**   dose dependent and another reason to limit
     E **True**   oestrogen dosage. Although there is evidence that
atherosclerosis in humans is associated with similar
changes the relationship of long term use of such
preparations is not clear.

Ref 19

2.108 A **True**   Decreased HDL cholesterol, decreased serum
     B **True**   albumin and a decreased carbohydrate tolerance
     C **True**   have occurred in most studies of the combined oral
     D **False**   contraceptive just as these changes occur in normal
     E **False**   pregnancy. There is a decreased serum anti Xa and
this decrease below 20% of normal has been used as
a screening test for patients susceptible to
thrombosis. There is no change in prolactin levels on
the pill.

Ref 19

2.109 A **False**   The unruptured luteinized follicle is probably a
     B **True**   common occurrence but can only be recognized by
     C **True**   the absence of an ovulation ostium or stigma at
     D **False**   laparoscopy as other endometrial and plasma
     E **True**   parameters of ovulation are normal. It is associated
with endometriosis and it may be that the decreased
steroid levels in the peritoneal fluid fail to inhibit the
growth of endometrial seedlings.

I A Brosens & P R Koninckx in Ref 3 Vol 1

2.110 A **False**   The dowager's hump of spinal osteoporosis, is the
     B **True**   result of oestrogen deficiency. Common side effects
     C **True**   of progestogens are acne, depression, mastalgia,
     D **True**   water retention and other symptoms of the
     E **False**   premenstrual syndrome. It is possible that the arterial
complications of the oral contraceptive is due to the
progestogen component, but 'pill cholestasis' is due
to the oestrogen component.

MacDonald in Ref 14

2.111 In anorexia nervosa in females
    A secondary amenorrhoea is a recognised feature
    B endogenous oestrogen levels are low
    C follicle stimulating hormone (FSH) levels are high
    D is associated with lanugo hair
    E marriage leads to improvement

2.112 The effectiveness of oral contraception is reduced following interaction with
    A Ampicillin
    B Vitamin B12
    C Phenobarbitone
    D Phenytoin
    E Thyroxine

2.113 Premature menopause is associated with
    A pernicious anaemia
    B chromosomal abnormalities
    C radiotherapy
    D a positive family history
    E polycystic ovarian syndrome

2.114 The resistant ovary syndrome
    A can be diagnosed by ovarian biopsy
    B can be effectively treated by gonadotrophins
    C produces excess androgens
    D characteristically has a high plasma FSH
    E is intermittent

2.115 Congenital adrenal hyperplasia is associated with
    A stillbirth
    B precocious pseudo puberty in male infants
    C symptoms and signs of salt loss
    D neonatal jaundice
    E ambiguous genitalia in the newborn

(Answers overleaf)

2.111 A **True**   This is essentially a psychological disorder with
      B **True**   endocrine manifestations operating through
      C **False**   hypothalamic mediation. FSH and LH levels are low
      D **True**   with consequent low oestrogen levels and secondary
      E **False**   amenorrhoea. There is frequently a generalised
                      reappearance of lanugo hair. It is more common in
                      the higher social classes and marriage
                      institutionalizes the disorder, perpetuating it.

A H Crisp in Ref 13

2.112 A **True**   Barbiturates, phenytoin and carbamazadine are
      B **False**   powerful liver enzyme inducers which accelerate the
      C **True**   metabolism of the sex steroids in the liver resulting
      D **True**   in contraceptive failure in low dose combined pills.
      E **False**   Two low-dose OC pills will usually overcome this. It
                      is generally believed that ampicillin diminishes the
                      absorption of steroids.

Ref 19

2.113 A **True**   Premature menopause usually defined as ovarian
      B **True**   failure before 35 years of age may be due to surgical
      C **True**   or radiotherapeutic ablation of the ovaries. It may be
      D **True**   familial women with mosaicism (45X/46XX) and
      E **False**   Triple X females (47XXX) may have such a
                      menopause. A screen for auto antibodies should be
                      performed because an auto immune basis is
                      suspected and pernicious anaemia, hypothyroidism
                      and Addisons disease may be associated.

D A Davey in Ref 4

2.114 A **False**   The resistant ovary syndrome is a rare variant of
      B **False**   primary ovarian failure distinguished by intermittent
      C **False**   resolution of the failure and normalisation of the FSH
      D **True**   levels. It is untreatable, will not respond to
      E **True**   exogenous gonadotrophins and cannot (and should
                      not) be diagnosed by an ovarian biopsy.

M Hull in Ref 3 Vol 2

2.115 A **False**   Congenital adrenal hyperplasia, most commonly due
      B **True**   to 21 hydroxylase deficiency causes increased
      C **True**   synthesis of androgens leading to ambiguous
      D **False**   genitalia in female neonates and precocious pseudo
      E **True**   puberty in male infants. Because of the defective
                      synthesis of aldosterone sodium loss occurs. The
                      basic defect is a block of aldosterone and cortisol
                      synthesis with precursors being diverted to the
                      synthesis of androgens.

J D Bailey in Ref 13

2.116 Severe hyperstimulation syndrome associated with human menopausal gonadotrophin therapy may be manifested clinically by:
A abdominal pain
B ascites
C hypovolaemic shock
D follicular cysts
E thrombo-embolic episodes

2.117 The following results found in a 35 year old normally menstruating woman are normal:
A plasma testosterone 4 nmols/1
B plasma FSH 7 IU/l
C oestradiol 50 pmol/l
D progesterone 30 nmol/l
E prolactin 300 mu/l

2.118 Which of the following statements are true?
A rifampicin is associated with oral contraceptive failure
B methyldopa occasionally causes folic acid deficiency anaemia
C the SLE syndrome, associated with long-term hydrallazine therapy is reversible on stopping treatment
D clindamycin and Lincomycin are associated with fatal necrotising colitis
E methyldopa causes lethargy and drowsiness

2.119 Polycystic ovary syndrome
A should be diagnosed by laparoscopy
B should be treated by wedge resection
C produces hypoestrogenism
D has both negative and positive feedback mechanisms intact
E is best treated by clomiphene

(*Answers overleaf*)

2.116 A **True**   Hyperstimulation syndrome is a severe complication
      B **True**   of treatment manifested by marked ovarian
      C **True**   enlargement, ascites, hypovolaemic shock and
      D **False**   implied changes in distribution of body fluids. The
      E **True**   bilateral ovarian enlargement is due to theca lutein
                      cyst formation. This may also cause hyperviscosity
                      and thrombo-embolic episodes. Treatment is
                      conservative and supportive, but with proper
                      supervision of therapy the syndrome should not
                      occur.

R R Shearman in Ref 3 Vol 3

2.117 A **False**   The units used are those recommended by WHO and
      B **True**   widely used throughout the world, although there are
      C **False**   exceptions in various laboratories, principally in the
      D **True**   United States.
      E **True**   The normal range of values in this woman would be:

FSH	1–10 IU/l
LH	1–50 IU/l
Prolactin	50–800 mu/l
Oestradiol	100–1000 pmol/l
Progesterone	0.5–40 nmol/l
Testosterone	0.5–2 nmol/l

2.118 A **True**   It is important to know the drug interactions and side
      B **False**   effects that occur with drugs commonly used in
      C **True**   obstetrics and gynaecology.
      D **True**
      E **True**

2.119 A **False**   Although polycystic ovary disease has a typical
      B **False**   appearance, there is no advantage in performing a
      C **False**   laparoscopy. Excessive androgen production and
      D **True**   hirsutism is an essential feature but the former is
      E **True**   difficult to detect by routine laboratory methods.
                      Treatment is by Clomiphene, but glucocorticoid
                      therapy is the best alternative or adjunct to
                      Clomiphene if there is adrenal hyperandrogenism
                      because it may reduce the high associated abortion
                      rate. Ovarian wedge resection produces fimbrial
                      adhesions and has little place in management.

M Hull in Ref 3 Vol 2

2.120 The following drugs are known to cause hyperprolactinaemia:
A   metoclopramide (Maxolon)
B   cimetidine (Tagamet)
C   chlorpromazine (Largactil)
D   methyldopa (Aldomet)
E   chlorthalidone (Hygroton)

2.121 Injectable progestogens used for contraceptive purposes
A   include medroxyprogesterone acetate
B   cause irregular vaginal bleeding
C   cause amenorrhoea
D   carry a risk of venous thrombosis
E   cause hypertension

2.122 Progestogen only contraception
A   has a lesser effect on hepatic function than the combined oral contraceptive pill
B   causes HDL levels to rise
C   produces headaches less commonly than the combined oral contraceptive
D   by intramuscular injection causes amenorrhoea in approximately 30% of patients
E   taken orally has a 19 hour duration of effectiveness

2.123 The following metabolic effects occur with oestrogen administration:
A   decreased aldosterone production
B   increased TBG
C   increased plasma renin activity
D   increased serum albumin concentration
E   increased glucose tolerance

(Answers overleaf)

2.120 A **True**   The most common cause of galactorrhoea is drugs,
       B **True**   and these include metoclopramide, methyldopa,
       C **True**   phenothiazines such as chlorpromazine and the oral
       D **True**   contraceptive pill. Psychiatric patients may well be
       E **False**   prescribed phenothiazines. Digoxin does cause
                      hyperprolactinaemia, chlorthalidone does not. The H_2
                      receptor antagonist cimetidine also causes this
                      complication.

Ref 25

2.121 A **True**   The advantages of injectable progestogens as
       B **True**   contraceptives is that they are given every 3–6
       C **True**   months and that they do not produce the metabolic
       D **False**   complications of oestrogen therapy. However the
       E **False**   high incidence of irregular bleeding and
                      amenorrhoea make them unpopular. They are
                      specifically recommended (and licensed) in patients
                      whose partners have just had a vasectomy (until the
                      sperm count falls) and in women who have had
                      recent rubella immunization.

M Elstein in Ref 3 Vol 2

2.122 A **True**   Progestogen contraception has a smaller effect upon
       B **False**   clotting, glucose tolerance or liver function than the
       C **True**   combined oral contraception, but decreases HDL. The
       D **True**   short duration of action necessitates that the pill is
       E **True**   taken at the same time each day. Although
                      intramuscular depot Medroxyprogesterone and
                      Norethisterone acetate commonly produces
                      amenorrhoea the pregnancy rates 18 months after
                      cessation of this means of contraception is the same
                      as following discontinuation of the coil or the
                      combined oral contraceptive.

M Elstein Ref 3 Vol 2

2.123 A **False**   Oestrogen produces increased aldosterone
       B **True**   production and increased levels of TBG-PBI.
       C **True**   Angiotensinogen and plasma renin activity are also
       D **False**   increased. The principal effects on serum proteins
       E **False**   are a decrease in serum albumin and haptoglobulins
                      and a marked increase in caeruloplasmin. Glucose
                      tolerance is impaired.

MacDonald in Ref 14

2.124 The following statements about LH-RH analogues are correct:
A   LH-RH agonists are contraceptive
B   LH-RH agonists are administered by nasal spray
C   LH-RH analogues are contraceptive in humans
D   LH-RH is a steroid
E   LH-RH analogues are useful in the treatment of infertility

2.125 A negative progestrogen challenge test
A   suggests low endogenous oestrogen levels
B   indicates that clomiphene is a suitable drug to induce ovulation
C   would be expected in cases of primary ovarian failure
D   would be expected in amenorrhoea associated with anorexia nervosa
E   is typical of hyperprolactinaemic amenorrhoea

2.126 Human menopausal gonadotrophin (HMG or Pergonal) therapy for infertility
A   is associated with an increased incidence of identical twins
B   is taken orally
C   requires careful monitoring of FSH levels
D   requires a mid cycle injection of human chorionic gonadotrophin (HCG)
E   causes a hyperstimulation syndrome

2.127 Primary hypothyroidism is associated with
A   amenorrhoea
B   infertility
C   increased fetal wastage
D   elevated thyroid stimulating hormone levels (TSH)
E   exaggerated ankle jerk

(*Answers overleaf*)

2.124 A **True**   LH-RH is a decapeptide which has not fulfilled its
       B **True**   theoretical possibility of use in infertility. The
       C **False** inhibitory analogues are not powerful enough for
       D **False** contraceptive use in humans. Strangely, it is the
       E **False** agonists which have a marked anti-reproductive
                    effect following chronic administration by a nasal
                    spray.

S Nillius in Ref 3 Vol 2

2.125 A **True**   The administration of a progestogen (e.g.
       B **False** Medroxyprogesterone acetate 5 mg daily for five
       C **True**   days) will only precipitate vaginal bleeding in
       D **True**   subjects who have adequate levels of endogenous
       E **True**   oestrogens. Subjects with primary ovarian failure
                    and anorexia will almost certainly have negative
                    tests. Hyperprolactinaemia is associated with
                    oestrogen deficiency and is associated with a
                    negative test. This test is a reasonable screening
                    procedure to distinguish between serious and benign
                    causes of amenorrhoea and also if positive indicates
                    which subjects should respond to Clomiphene.

H S Jacobs in Ref 25

2.126 A **False** HMG therapy should only be used in patients who
       B **False** have failed to respond to or do not fulfil the criteria
       C **False** for treatment with clomiphene. It has to be given in
       D **True**   several intra-muscular injections, requires an
       E **True**   injection of HCG to replace the LH surge, requires
                    biochemical monitoring of oestrogen levels to
                    minimise the risk of hyperstimulation syndrome. It is
                    also expensive! Such therapy is associated with an
                    increased incidence of non-identical multiple
                    pregnancies.

H S Jacobs in Ref 25

2.127 A **True**   Primary hypothyroidism, the commonest type
       B **True**   hypothyroidism, is associated with menorrhagia and
       C **True**   infertility. However amenorrhoea occurs in a
       D **True**   minority. Patients who do conceive have an
       E **False** increased rate of fetal loss. TSH levels are elevated
                    due to the negative feedback effect of depressed
                    thyroxine levels. The clinical picture is typical and
                    includes depressed tendon reflexes.

Ref 13

2.128 Congenital adrenal hyperplasia may be due to deficiency of the following enzymes involved in steroid biosynthesis:
  A   21-hydroxylase
  B   7-desmolase
  C   4-decarboxylase
  D   20-22 desmolase
  E   11-hydroxylase

2.129 Biochemical changes expected in congenital adrenal hyperplasia due to 21 hydroxylase deficiency include:
  A   increased urinary pregnanetriol
  B   increased urinary ketosteroids
  C   increased serum aldosterone
  D   decreased serum testosterone
  E   increased serum 17 hydroxyprogesterone

2.130 Clomiphene citrate (Clomid) used in the treatment of infertility
  A   is associated with ovarian cyst formation
  B   increases the risk of fetal malformation
  C   causes vasomotor symptoms as a side effect
  D   causes breast discomfort
  E   is prescribed in a starting dose of 500 mg daily for five days each month

2.131 Clomiphene citrate (Clomid) used in the treatment of infertility
  A   is a steroid molecule
  B   acts by direct stimulation of follicle stimulating hormone (FSH)
  C   has some anti-oestrogenic effect
  D   increases circulating oestrogen levels
  E   depends upon an intact positive feedback response of LH to oestrogens

(Answers overleaf)

2.128 A **True**   The commonest defect in congenital adrenal
       B **False**   hyperplasia is 21-hydroxylase. 20-22 desmolase
       C **False**   deficiency also occurs causing complete failure of
       D **True**   adrenal steroid synthesis in a phenotypic female as
       E **True**   the block is in the very early conversion.
                      11-hydroxylase deficiency also occurs and like
                      21-hydroxylase deficiency causes ambiguous
                      genitalia in female infants and precocious pseudo
                      puberty in male infants.

J D Bailey in Ref 13

2.129 A **True**   The 21 hydroxylase block causes its immediate
       B **True**   precursor 17 hydroxyprogesterone to accumulate
       C **False**   and diverts precursors to androgen synthesis causing
       D **False**   increased urinary pregnanetriol and ketosteroids and
       E **True**   increased serum testosterone. Aldosterone synthesis
                      is defective.

J D Bailey in Ref 13

2.130 A **True**   Clomiphene citrate is associated with ovarian cyst
       B **False**   formation and repeated prescriptions especially of
       C **True**   high doses demands pelvic examination. It may
       D **True**   cause vasomotor symptoms, breast discomfort,
       E **False**   visual symptoms and rarely alopecia. A large study
                      has demonstrated no association with fetal
                      malformation. The starting dose is 50 mg daily for
                      five days each month.

H S Jacobs in Ref 25

2.131 A **False**   Clomiphene citrate is a non-steroidal relative of
       B **False**   stilboestrol which acts by enhancing the FSH
       C **True**   response to low oestrogen levels by occupying
       D **True**   oestrogen receptors in the hypothalamus (requiring
       E **True**   intact negative feedback response). It acts by
                      restoring FSH levels which in turn increase
                      circulating oestrogens. However ovulation depends
                      upon an intact positive feedback response of LH to
                      the rising oestrogen levels. Clomiphene has some
                      anti-oestrogenic action and therefore should be used
                      in the lowest dose which restores ovulation.

H S Jacobs in Ref 25

2.132 The following statements concerning the hyperstimulation syndrome associated with the use of agents to induce ovulation are true:
A   there is a good correlation between the incidence of side effects and dosage
B   it may be avoided by withholding the mid cycle injection of HCG in the presence of high oestrogen levels
C   it occurs with Clomiphene
D   patients with polycystic ovaries before treatment are more likely to develop the syndrome
E   the incidence can be reduced by ultrasonic examination.

2.133 The clinical syndrome due to hyperprolactinaemia in the female characteristically includes:
A   amenorrhoea
B   headaches
C   dyspareunia
D   galactorrhoea in more than 60% of cases
E   scanty cervical mucus and curettings

2.134 Oligospermia is associated with
A   prolactinomas
B   small testes
C   Klinefelter's syndrome
D   testicular feminization
E   negative post coital test

2.135 The following tests are relevant in assessing male infertility:
A   follicle stimulating hormone
B   cystoscopy
C   seminal culture
D   testicular biopsy
E   plasma testosterone

(*Answers overleaf*)

2.132 A **False**   The severity of this potentially lethal complication of
     B **True**   Human Menopausal Gonadotrophin therapy does not
     C **False**   correlate well with dosage. This is not surprising
     D **True**   because of the widely varying individual response.
     E **True**   Pelvic examination should be performed to exclude
polycystic ovaries before treatment is started as
these patients are more likely to develop the
syndrome. It may be avoided by careful assessment
of follicular size by ultrasound or by plasma
oestrogens and withholding the HCG injection in the
event of excessive stimulation.

R P Shearman in Ref 3 Vol 3

2.133 A **True**   In the hyperprolactinaemic state there is usually
     B **False**   secondary amenorrhoea or oligomenorrhoea
     C **True**   although primary amenorrhoea may occur.
     D **False**   Headaches are unusual except in the small number of
     E **True**   patients who harbour a pituitary tumour.
Dyspareunia and loss of libido occur due to the
oestrogen deficient state which also explains
atrophic changes in the genital tract. Galactorrhoea
may be expected in about 30% of cases.

H S Jacobs in Ref 3 Vol 1

2.134 A **False**   Reduced numbers of sperm occur in men with small
     B **True**   testes and a common result is infertility with a
     C **False**   negative post coital test. Patients with testicular
     D **False**   feminization do not produce sperm and patients with
     E **True**   Klinefelter's syndrome are azoospermic.

J Pryor in Ref 3 Vol 4

2.135 A **True**   A high FSH frequently indicates testicular failure and
     B **False**   testicular biopsy will give useful information
     C **True**   concerning spermatogenesis. In patients with an
     D **True**   apparently good sperm count the spermatozoa are
     E **False**   less motile and healthy because of chronic infection
of the seminal fluid. Hence culture and a search for
the presence of white cells in the seminal fluid is
important.

J Pryor in Ref 3 Vol 4

2.136 The following endocrine findings characteristically occur in hyperprolactinaemia:
    A   low serum oestrogens
    B   a negative oestrogen provocation test
    C   a positive progestogen challenge test
    D   impaired short term pulsatility of luteinizing hormone (LH) secretion
    E   elevated follicle stimulating hormone levels (FSH)

2.137 When Bromocriptine is used in the treatment of hyperprolactinaemia
    A   the dose is 50 mg daily
    B   a skull X-ray should be performed annually
    C   hypotension is a side effect
    D   prolactin levels do not fall in patients with a pituitary tumour
    E   libido is increased

2.138 The following statements about prolactin secreting pituitary tumours are correct:
    A   they tend to cause higher prolactin levels than other causes of hyperprolactinaemia
    B   a lateral skull X-ray showing a normal pituitary fossa excludes the diagnosis
    C   they enlarge during pregnancy
    D   a progressive visual field defect suggests enlargement of the tumour
    E   suprasellar extension is an indication for primary surgical treatment

2.139 The ovary in polycystic ovarian syndrome characteristically shows
    A   theca cell hyperplasia
    B   granulosa cell hyperplasia
    C   increased fatty infiltration
    D   fibrosis
    E   capsular thickening

(*Answers overleaf*)

2.136 A **True**   Hyperprolactinaemia causes a disorder of
       B **True**   hypothalamia-pituitary control of FSH and LH
       C **False**   secretion which results in an oestrogen deficient
       D **True**   state. The progestogen challenge test is therefore
       E **False**   negative. There is no LH response to an oestrogen
                       challenge in mid cycle demonstrating a defective
                       positive feeback mechanism. Pulsatile release of LH
                       is impaired and FSH levels are not elevated. All these
                       abnormalities return to normal with treatment.

H S Jacobs in Ref 3 Vol 1

2.137 A **False**   The dose of Bromocriptine is 1.25 mg daily rising in
       B **False**   increments to 30 mg daily. Hypotension is a side
       C **True**   effect and libido may increase as ovulation returns
       D **False**   and the symptoms of oestrogen deficiency are
       E **True**   relieved. All patients should have X-rays of the
                       pituitary fossa before treatment to exclude a tumour
                       but they are not necessary annually. Prolactin levels
                       fall in patients with a prolactin secreting tumour.

H S Jacobs in Ref 3 Vol 1

2.138 A **True**   A very high prolactin level (greater than 2000 mu/l)
       B **False**   suggests a tumour as the cause. A lateral skull X-ray
       C **True**   is inadequate to demonstrate normality of the
       D **True**   pituitary fossa and in the presence of
       E **False**   hyperprolactinaemia tomography or cone views
                       should be performed. These tumours may be
                       sensitive to oestrogens and so may enlarge during
                       pregnancy. Enlargement may be suggested by a
                       progressive visual field defect and testing of the
                       fields should be performed during pregnancy.
                       Suprasellar extension was an indication for surgical
                       treatment, although use of Bromocriptine now
                       suggests that it is effective alone in reducing tumour
                       size as well as prolactin level.

H S Jacobs in Ref 3 Vol 1

2.139 A **True**   In this condition the ovary is often enlarged and
       B **False**   polycystic, the thecal cells being hyperplastic and the
       C **False**   granulosa cells atretic.
       D **False**
       E **True**

D T Baird in Ref 25

2.140 The following are characteristic endocrine findings in polycystic ovarian syndrome:
A   increased plasma androstenedione
B   increased testosterone production rate
C   increased basal luteinizing hormone (LH)
D   increased plasma follicle stimulating hormone (FSH)
E   reduced urinary oestrogen excretion

2.141 Androstenedione is secreted in the normal female by
A   the ovaries
B   the liver
C   the adrenal glands
D   peripheral adipose tissue
E   the pancreas

2.142 Sex hormone binding globulin (SHBG)
A   is produced by the ovary
B   is depressed in hyperthyroidism
C   is increased by increasing levels of plasma androgens
D   is depressed by increasing plasma oestrogens
E   is increased in pregnancy

2.143 The following substances are potent androgens in the normal female:
A   testosterone
B   androstenedione
C   dehydro-epiandrosterone (DHEA)
D   dihydrotestosterone
E   androstenediol

2.144 Benign idiopathic hirsutism may be successfully treated by the following methods:
A   a combined oestrogen and progestogen oral contraceptive pill
B   oxytetracycline
C   cyproterone acetate
D   prednisolone
E   electrolysis

(*Answers overleaf*)

2.140 A **True**   The hyperplastic theca cells in this condition lead to
       B **True**   increased production of androstenedione and
       C **True**   therefore testosterone. Luteinizing hormone is
       D **False**   characteristically increased but does not surge in mid
       E **False**   cycle to stimulate ovulation. FSH is low and the
granulosa cells atretic, but oestrogens are produced
by peripheral conversion of androstenedione
maintaining an oestrogenized state.

D T Baird in Ref 25

2.141 A **True**   Androstenedione, the main androgen precursor, is
       B **False**   secreted by the adrenal glands and the ovaries. It is
       C **True**   converted in peripheral adipose tissue to active
       D **False**   androgens.
       E **False**

Ref 25

2.142 A **False**   SHBG is a globulin of molecular weight 52000
       B **False**   produced by the liver. It is increased by elevated
       C **False**   plasma oestrogen levels, pregnancy and
       D **False**   hyperthyroidism, and decreases after the
       E **True**   menopause. It is also depressed by increasing
plasma androgens thereby producing a vicious circle
in hirsutism by increasing the amount of 'active' or
non bound testosterone available.

A Decherney Ref 3 Vol 1

2.143 A **True**   Androstenedione is a weak androgen and is the main
       B **False**   precursor of Testosterone. Dehydro-epiandrosterone
       C **False**   is an extremely weak androgen secreted by the
       D **True**   adrenal glands and is a precursor of negligible
       E **True**   amounts of androstenedione and testosterone. Its
assay is a useful measure of adrenal/androgen
function and indeed more Testosterone is produced
by this peripheral conversion than by glandular
secretion.

A Decherney in Ref 3 Vol 1

2.144 A **True**   Many drugs have been used to treat hirsutism, but
       B **False**   combined oral contraceptives have fewest side
       C **True**   effects. They have to be prescribed for several
       D **True**   months. Cyproterone acetate is the most effective
       E **True**   working at the level of the hair follicle as an anti-
androgen and also decreasing gonadotrophin
production.

A Decherney Ref 3 Vol 1

2.145 Biochemical changes in idiopathic (benign) hirsutism often include
A   raised plasma testosterone
B   raised testosterone production rate
B   raised testosterone metabolic clearance rate
D   normal plasma androstenedione
E   raised plasma free testosterone

2.146 In the treatment of hirsutism
A   dexamethasone is used when there is an adrenal cause
B   skin irradiation is justified for severe cases
C   cyproterone acetate causes acne
D   cyproterone acetate causes loss of libido
E   cyproterone acetate is an oestrogen

2.147 Primary hypothalamic failure
A   is diagnosed by gonadotrophin deficiency
B   is diagnosed by low serum LHRH
C   is associated with anosmia
D   is associated with Sheehan's syndrome
E   is associated with 'the tall girl' syndrome

2.148 Luteal phase deficiency
A   follows defective follicular maturation
B   has inadequate luteal progesterone production
C   is corrected by HCG
D   is associated with delayed menstruation
E   is associated with hyperprolactinaemia

2.149 Osteoporosis
A   is less common in black than white women
B   occurs no more commonly in patients with Turner's syndrome
C   occurs after the menopause because calcium is lost from the skeleton at the rate of approximately 1% per year
D   is prevented by oestrogens
E   produces fractures in 30% of 70 year old women

(*Answers overleaf*)

2.145 A **False**   Testosterone production is increased in this
       B **True**   condition but the proportion of testosterone bound to
       C **True**   sex hormone binding globulin is reduced. There is
       D **False**   also increased conversion of testosterone to
       E **True**   dihydrotestosterone by the hair follicles. Plasma
                       androstenedione is elevated.

A Decherney in Ref 3 Vol 1

2.146 A **True**   Dexamethasone is effective therapy for adrenal
       B **False**   causes of hirsutism and oral contraceptives for
       C **True**   ovarian causes. Cyproterone is a progestogen which
       D **True**   causes loss of libido and acne and is therefore best
       E **False**   used with cyclical oestrogens. Irradiation is neither
                       helpful nor safe although it has been used in the past.

H S Jacobs in Ref 25

2.147 A **False**   Gonadotrophin deficiency may be due to
       B **False**   hypothalamic or pituitary failure and an assay for
       C **True**   LHRH does not yet exist. Kallmans syndrome is the
       D **False**   association of hypothalamic failure and anosmia. The
       E **False**   tall girl syndrome is constitutional and is not
                       associated with amenorrhoea.

M Hull in Ref 3 Vol 2

2.148 A **True**   Luteal phase deficiency is defined by inadequate
       B **True**   luteal progesterone production and is due to a
       C **False**   defective follicular phase. All treatment is
       D **False**   disappointing, but HCG alone does not help. It is
       E **False**   associated with a short rather than a prolonged luteal
                       phase and not with hyperprolactinaemia, which
                       usually leads to amenorrhoea.

Ref 25

2.149 A **True**   Postmenopausal osteoporosis occurs in trabecular
       B **False**   bone; the vertebral bodies, upper femur and lower
       C **True**   radius, and fractures of one or more of these bones
       D **True**   occurred in 30% of patients aged 70. It is less common
       E **True**   in black patients and in women who undergo regular or
                       strenuous exercise. Oestrogen therapy does prevent
                       loss of calcium at the rate of 1% per year, but this
                       calcium loss may be increased when oestrogen therapy
                       is eventually discontinued.

D McKay Hart in Ref 3 Vol 2

2.150 Progestogen only contraceptive pills
   A   act by suppressing ovulation
   B   have a higher failure rate than combined oral contraceptives
   C   cause intermenstrual bleeding
   D   are taken continuously
   E   are composed of 11 alpha OH progesterone derivatives

2.151 The following are associated with the increased risk of thrombosis in women taking combined oral contraceptives:
   A   increased platelet adhesiveness
   B   increased clotting factor VII
   C   increased antithrombin III
   D   increased clotting factor X
   E   decreased plasminogen

2.152 The following intra-uterine contraceptive devices are approved for general use in Britain at this time:
   A   copper 7
   B   Dalkon Shield
   C   Grafenberg ring
   D   Lippes loop
   E   progestasert

2.153 A Lippes loop intra-uterine contraceptive device
   A   is available in four different sizes
   B   is radio opaque
   C   contains copper which has a contraceptive effect
   D   often exacerbates menorrhagia
   E   has a failure rate of about 0.3/100 woman years

2.154 The progestogenic side effects of oral contraception include
   A   heavy menstrual flow
   B   fluid retention
   C   tiredness
   D   reduced libido
   E   vaginal discharge

(Answers overleaf)

2.150 A **False**   They do not suppress ovulation and therefore have a
     B **True**   higher failure rate. They often cause intermenstrual
     C **True**   bleeding, are taken continuously and contain either
     D **True**   17 alpha OH progesterone derivatives or 19
     E **False**   nortestosterone derivatives.

M Elstein in Ref 3 Vol 2

2.151 A **False**   The incidence of thromboembolism in patients taking
     B **True**   combined oral contraceptives is thought to be related
     C **False**   to the dose of oestrogens. 30 ug ethinyl oestradiol
     D **True**   daily is now the recommended dose. Changes in
     E **False**   platelets are not considered to be a significant factor
but there are changes in both clotting system and
fibrinolytic system which are interdependent. Factor
VII and factor X are elevated and antithrombin III
reduced. Fibrinolysis is also increased and
plasmin produced by conversion of fibrinogen.

Ref 19

2.152 A **True**   The Dalkon shield has been withdrawn from use
     B **False**   because of reports from America linking its use with
     C **False**   intra-uterine infection, septicaemia and death. The
     D **True**   Grafenberg ring, a rather old device, is not
     E **False**   recommended because passage of the ring into the
peritoneal cavity has been associated with serious
damage to bowel. The progestogen-loaded device,
Progestasert, has been withdrawn because of
reports associating its use with an increased
incidence of ectopic pregnancy.

Ref 19

2.153 A **True**   Lippes loops are tailored to fit different sizes of
     B **True**   uterine cavities and are radio opaque. They are
     C **False**   classified as inert devices, not containing copper.
     D **True**   They have a failure rate higher than oral
     E **True**   contraceptive pills but lower than other methods of
contraception. Like all intra-uterine devices they often
exacerbate menorrhagia.

Ref 19

2.154 A **False**   In general the side effects of oral contraceptives can
     B **False**   be identified as predominantly oestrogenic or
     C **True**   progestogenic. Oestrogenic side effects include
     D **True**   nausea, fluid retention, increased menstrual flow and
     E **False**   vaginal discharge. Tiredness, depression, acne,
vaginal dryness and reduced libido are probably
progestogenic.

R MacDonald in Ref 14

2.155 The following statements about prostaglandins are appropriate:
A   Amniotic fluid levels of prostaglandin E_2 and F_2 alpha increase in late pregnancy
B   During spontaneous labour amniotic fluid prostaglandins bear little relationship to the progress of labour
C   Cholesterol is the main precursor
D   The production of prostaglandin is decreased by the ingestion of aspirin
E   Prostaglandin levels in amniotic fluid do not increase during oxytocin-induced labour.

2.156 Progesterone
A   is secreted by the adrenal cortex
B   produces respiratory acidosis
C   increases growth of endometrial cilia
D   is anabolic
E   reduces urinary excretion of sodium

2.157 Carcinoma of the vulva
A   has a five year survival of 40–50%
B   is less common in orthodox Muslims
C   is Stage II if the tumour is greater than 2 cm in diameter without palpable enlarged inguinal nodes
D   with a positive Cloquet node suggests deep external iliac involvement
E   recurrence after radical vulvectomy should be treated by radiotherapy

2.158 Clear cell adenocarcinoma of the vagina in Diethylstilboestrol exposed females
A   occurs in approximately 1–5% of exposed females
B   is more common if DES exposure occurs in mid-trimester pregnancy
C   has a five-year actuarial survival of over 70%
D   involves the cervix in 40% of cases
E   may have false negative vaginal cytology in 20% of cases

(*Answers overleaf*)

2.155 A **True**   Amniotic fluid levels of PGE$_2$ and F$_2$ alpha increase in
       B **False**   late pregnancy, during spontaneous labour and
       C **False**   induced labour during the acceleration phase. The
       D **True**   levels increase with progress of labour. Ingestion of
       E **False**   aspirin prevents the conversion of prostaglandin
                       from arachidonic acid and its main precursor.

S Karim in Ref 14

2.156 A **True**   Progesterone is produced and secreted by the
       B **False**   adrenal cortex, ovary and placenta. It stimulates the
       C **False**   respiratory centre producing hyperventilation,
       D **False**   respiratory alkalosis and hence maintenance of pH by
       E **True**   urinary excretion of bicarbonate and sodium. It
                       produces breast alveolar growth, smooth muscle
                       relaxation, a slight rise in body temperature and
                       controls the endometrial proliferative effect of
                       oestrogen. Growth of endometrial cilia and microvilli
                       are increased by oestrogens and reversed by
                       progestogens.

MacDonald in Ref 14

2.157 A **False**   Vulval malignancy is usually a squamous carcinoma
       B **True**   with a five year survival of 60–70%. It is common
       C **True**   among the poor with bad hygiene and is less
       D **True**   frequently found in orthodox Muslims. The complex
       E **False**   classification is based upon the size of the primary
                       and the presence of nodes or distant secondaries.
                       Recurrence following radical vulvectomy is usually
                       treated with further surgery.

H R Barber in Ref 26

2.158 A **False**   Clear cell adenocarcinoma occurs in less than 0.1% of
       B **False**   exposed females with the maximum risk occuring
       C **True**   early in pregnancy and is very slight after the 16th
       D **True**   week. The 5-year survival rate is 78%. False vaginal
       E **True**   cytology is common due to the difficulty of
                       differentiating tumour cells from endometrial cells.

S Robboy in Ref 3

2.159 Botryoide sarcoma in childhood
A   is less common than benign lower genital polyps in childhood
B   is a mixed mesodermal tumour
C   is sensitive to chemotherapy
D   frequently requires radical surgery
E   has a characteristically malignant histology

2.160 Carcinoma of the vagina is more common with the following conditions:
A   post-menopausal oestrogen therapy
B   herpes
C   use of the ring pessary
D   testicular feminization
E   high parity

2.161 The following statements about ovarian carcinoma are appropriate:
A   The five year survival for Stage IB disease is less than 60%
B   Endometriosis is observed in 25% of cases of clear cell (mesonephroid) tumours
C   Scandinavian women have a low incidence of ovarian malignancies
D   Positive paraaortic nodes are found in 10–15% of cases in Stage I disease
E   To stage ovarian malignancies accurately an examination under anaesthetic (EUA) is often necessary.

2.162 Endodermal sinus tumour of the ovary
A   is an extra-embryonic tumour
B   occurs in teenage girls
C   secretes alpha feto protein
D   is a derivative of yolk sac endoderm
E   has a poor prognosis

(*Answers overleaf*)

2.159 A **False**
      B **False**
      C **True**
      D **True**
      E **False**

Botryoide sarcoma presents like a simple polyp but although rare is more common than a benign vaginal polyp. It used to be considered to be of mixed mesodermal origin, but it is now established to be a rhabdomyosarcoma. The histology is notoriously difficult, as malignant characteristics may not be clearly apparent. The poor prognosis of earlier years has been much improved by chemotherapy often combined with radical surgery and radiotherapy.

J Dewhurst in Ref 3

2.160 A **False**
      B **False**
      C **True**
      D **False**
      E **False**

Squamous carcinoma of the vagina is found in the post-menopausal woman. Long standing foreign bodies are a predisposing factor. Adenocarcinoma may follow exposure to DES in utero and also (rarely) in the site of septal endometriosis.

R M Feroze in Ref 4

2.161 A **True**
      B **True**
      C **False**
      D **True**
      E **False**

The five year survival for Stage IB disease is approximately 45%. The staging of ovarian malignancy is surgical and not clinical, and therefore an EUA is unhelpful. Staging laparotomy is mandatory. Positive para-aortic nodes are found in 12% of apparent Stage I cases. Scandinavian women have a very high incidence of carcinoma of the ovary and pelvic endometriosis occurs in more than 25% of cases of mesonephroid tumours in contrast to overall association with ovarian cancer of 8%

P Kolstad in Ref 27

2.162 A **True**
      B **True**
      C **True**
      D **True**
      E **False**

This extra-embryonic tumour is uncommon but one of the malignant tumours affecting young girls. It is often mixed with a dysgerminoma and the endodermal sinus cells secrete alpha feto protein and sometimes HCG. These are biochemical markers which greatly facilitate effective treatment. Until recently it had an appalling prognosis but now aggressive treatment with surgery and the newer cytotoxic agents have changed this and an improved survival rate can be anticipated.

R Begent in Ref 3 Vol 3

2.163 Types of tumour marker substances
  A are used in the treatment of hydatidiform mole
  B are used in the treatment of endodermal sinus tumour
  C are used in the treatment of mesonephric ovarian tumour
  D include alpha feto protein
  E include beta sub-unit HCG

2.164 Endometrial cancer associated with exogenous oestrogen therapy
  A occurs 5 to 10 times more commonly than in non-users
  B has the same overall prognosis as the tumour in non-users
  C is associated with adeno-acanthoma more than any other type
  D is less common than the overall national incidence if the oestrogen is in the form of the sequential oral contraceptive
  E has also been reported to be increased if oestrogen therapy is 'opposed' by 7 days of progestogen

2.165 Carcinoma of the endometrum
  A has an overall five-year survival of approximately 50%
  B if associated with oestrogen taking has a worse overall prognosis
  C is associated with extra-glandular conversion of oestrogens into androstenedione in the fat
  D Stage I is sub-divided according to histology
  E can be diagnozed by cytology as effectively as by an out-patient curettage

2.166 The following statements about radical vulvectomy are appropriate:
  A Lymphoedema of the legs is a persistent complication in 50% of cases.
  B The femoral artery is identified lateral to the femoral vein in the femoral triangle.
  C Cloquet's node is identified as the inferior node in the deep femoral group.
  D If the clitoris is involved, pelvic lymphadenectomy should always be performed.
  E The lower third of the urethra may be removed without affecting urinary continence.

(Answers overleaf)

2.163 A **True**   One of the most important advances in oncology has
      B **True**   been the recognition of specific marker substances
      C **False**   secreted by tumour cells. Unfortunately only a small
      D **True**   number of tumours have been recognized to secrete
      E **True**   such markers which are used in assessment of
                             effective therapy. Trophoblastic tumours secrete beta
                             sub-unit HCG and endodermal sinus tumours secrete
                             alpha feto protein.

C N Hudson in Ref 3 Vol 2

2.164 A **True**   The reported increased incidence of carcinoma of the
      B **False**   endometrium in oestrogen takers is convincing, but
      C **True**   most tumours are Stage I, Grade I with a five-year
      D **False**   survival of 95%–100%. Adenoacanthoma is the most
      E **False**   common tumour type. The tumour is less common
                             with the combined oral contraceptive because of the
                             protective effect of continuous progestogen and is
                             found more commonly in young girls taking the
                             sequential pill than the combined preparation. Seven
                             to thirteen days progestogen is protective against
                             hyperplasia and probably carcinoma.

J W W Studd & M H Thom in Ref 3 Vol 1

2.165 A **False**   Carcinoma of the endometrium has a 60%–65%
      B **False**   overall survival rate which is greater in oestrogen
      C **False**   takers as the majority are Stage I, Grade I with a
      D **True**   95%–100% five-year survival rate. It is much more
      E **False**   common with prolonged oestrogen therapy and
                             disorders of ovulation — theca cell tumours and fat
                             women where oestrone and oestradiol are produced
                             from adrenal androstenedione. Although currently
                             debated, it is unlikely that any cytology screening is
                             as useful as a study of tissue obtained from
                             endometrial biopsy.

J W W Studd & M H Thom in Ref 3 Vol 1

2.166 A **False**   Lymphoedema occurs in 5%–10% of cases, is usually
      B **True**   not severe and is transient. The femoral triangle
      C **True**   should be opened and the femoral vessels cleared of
      D **False**   lymphatic tissue. Cloquet's node is located just below
      E **True**   Poupart's ligament, and if positive for tumour
                             indicates the need for deep iliac node dissection.
                             Although lymphatics from the clitoris direct to the
                             pelvic nodes are described it is unusual to find pelvic
                             node metastases without disease in the inguinal
                             lymph nodes and therefore the condition of Cloquet's
                             node remains important.

P J Krupp in Ref 27

2.167 Carcinoma of the vulva
- **A** is increasing in incidence
- **B** is usually multifocal
- **C** is not related to parity
- **D** has a lymphatic spread primarily to the superficial inguinal nodes
- **E** is uncommon in black patients

2.168 Endometrioid carcinoma of the ovary
- **A** is a secondary lesion
- **B** accounts for 10–25% of ovarian adenocarcinoma
- **C** has a low incidence in black women
- **D** rarely contain clear cells
- **E** usually occurs in premenopausal patients

2.169 Serous cystadenocarcinoma
- **A** is the commonest malignant ovarian tumour
- **B** frequently contains psammoma bodies
- **C** is bilateral in less than 20% of cases
- **D** if ruptured, may cause pseudomyxoma peritoneii
- **E** presents most commonly as Stage III disease

2.170 In the treatment of ovarian cancer
- **A** whole pelvis irradiation is a useful adjunct to surgery in Stage III disease
- **B** second line chemotherapy frequently produces dramatic responses in previously resistant tumours
- **C** alkylating agents are cytotoxic throughout all phases of the cell cycle
- **D** the moving strip technique of whole abdomen irradiation takes six weeks to deliver the total dose
- **E** cells in the resting phase of the replication cycle are particularly vulnerable to the effects of chemo-therapeutic agents

(Answers overleaf)

2.167 A **True**   The increased incidence from 5% to 8% of all
     B **False**   gynaecological malignancies has been reported and
     C **True**   attributed largely to a rise in female life expenctancy.
     D **True**   Apart from the unusual so-called 'kiss lesions'
     E **False**   carcinoma of the vulva is usually unifocal. There is no
relationship with parity. The superficial inguinal
nodes are the primary nodal group for lymphatic
drainage. It is very much more common in black
patients.

Ref 26

2.168 A **False**   Endometrioid carcinoma is a common primary
     B **True**   epithelial tumour (15%). Its origin may be
     C **True**   endometriotic (hence its very low incidence in black
     D **False**   patients), or from metaplasia of pelvic mesothelium.
     E **False**   The patients are usually post menopausal and often
nulliparous. The frequent occurrence of clear cells
supports the assumption that these neoplasms are
mullerian in origin.

Ref 20

2.169 A **True**   Serous cystadenocarcinoma accounts for 50% of all
     B **True**   epithelial malignancies and is the most common
     C **False**   ovarian cancer in the adult female. Psammoma
     D **False**   bodies are encountered in approximately 30% of
     E **True**   serous tumours. Bilateral involvement occurs in
30–50% of cases. Pseudomyxoma peritoneii
complicates rupture of mucinous cysts. Tumour
spread has progressed to Stage III disease at the time
of presentation in approximately 50% of cases.

Ref 26

2.170 A **False**   Stage III disease has spread beyond the pelvis, and
     B **False**   therefore irradiation of the pelvis is of no value.
     C **True**   Whole abdomen irradiation is often useful and the
     D **False**   dose of approximately 2250 rads can be achieved in
     E **False**   twelve days by the moving strip technique. Second
line chemotherapy is usually disappointing.
Alkylating agents are cycle non-specific drugs and
cells in the active phase of replication are more
sensitive to the effects of cytotoxic drugs than those
in the resting phase.

P J Disaia in Ref 28

2.171 The following statements are true of borderline ovarian tumours:
  A   they are recognized most frequently in mucinous tumours
  B   there is no stromal invasion
  C   the 10-year survival rate is in excess of 90%
  D   50% of patients with borderline tumours die of the disease
  E   occur more commonly in the younger age groups

2.172 The following ovarian tumours are of germ-cell origin:
  A   Brenner tumour
  B   arrhenoblastoma
  C   dysgerminoma
  D   embryonal cell carcinoma
  E   yolk sac tumours

2.173 The following statements about germ cell tumours of the ovary are appropriate:
  A   gonadoblastomas usually occur in genetically abnormal individuals
  B   struma ovarii often presents with concomitant hypothyroidism
  C   chorio carcinoma may occur in nulligravid young women
  D   dysgerminomas occur predominantly in post menopausal women
  E   the most frequent complication of a mature cystic teratoma is torsion

2.174 The FIGO classification of carcinoma of the ovary
  A   is divided into I–V Stages
  B   is Stage II or more if ascites is present
  C   is Stage Ic if the tumour is limited to both ovaries
  D   is at least Stage III if peritoneal seedlings are present
  E   does not consider capsular invasion

(*Answers overleaf*)

2.171 A **False**   Although recognized in a wide range of ovarian
B **True**   tumours, border-line tumours which are also known
C **True**   as proliferative cystadenomas or tumours of low
D **True**   malignant potential are most commonly reported in
E **True**   serous tumours. The malignant histological
characteristics are confined to the surface epithelium.
Although the initial prognosis is excellent close
follow up of these patients is advocated in several
reports which demonstrate late recurrence.
Borderline tumours usually present as early stage
disease in young women.

W R Hart in Ref 28

2.172 A **False**   The importance of this rare group of solid tumours is
B **False**   that there have been striking advances in the results
C **True**   of chemotherapy because of the high synthetic index
D **True**   of these tumours and that many produce onco-fetal
E **True**   antigens which may be used as tumour markers.
Examples of tumours of germ-cell origin,
dysgerminoma, embryonal cell carcinoma,
non-gestational choriocarcinoma, teratoma,
polyembryoma, teratomas and the yolk sac tumours,
endodermal sinus or Teilum tumours.

H Fox & F A Langley in Ref 29

2.173 A **True**   Most germ cell tumours occur in young women and
B **False**   non-gestational choriocarcinoma may occur in
C **True**   children. Gonadoblastomas occur almost exclusively
D **False**   co-existant with abnormal genotype and 90% of
E **True**   cases are sex chromatin negative. Struma ovarii are
composed of thyroid parenchyma and approximately
30% of cases have clinical hyperthyroidism. Torsion
is the most common complication of dermoid cyst
(16%) and is much more frequent than either rupture
(1%) or malignant change (1%).

H Fox & F A Langley in Ref 29

2.174 'A **False**   Carcinoma of the ovary is divided into Stages I to IV,
B **False**   but there are numerous sub-stages of Stage I and
C **False**   Stage II. The tumour may be Stage I if ascites are
D **True**   present; will be Stage Ib if the tumour is limited to
E **False**   both ovaries, and peritoneal seedlings would indicate
Stage III. The classification does consider capsular
invasion as a sub-group. Fundamental to current
concepts of treatment of the cancer is protocol
staging to ensure the correct therapy relating to
chemotherapy particularly for Stages I and II.

R M Feroze in Ref 4

2.175 The following statements concerning ovarian cancer are correct:
A it is usually diagnozed correctly pre-operatively in approximately 50% of cases
B stage I is bilateral in 10–20% of cases
C stage I carcinoma of the ovary should not be operated on through a Pfannenstiel incision
D cancer cells in peritoneal washings indicate a Stage II disease
E unilateral Stage I ovarian cancer in a young woman should be treated by unilateral oophorectomy

2.176 The following conditions are associated with ovarian tumours:
A thrombophlebitis migrans
B mixed mesodermal tumours
C Peutz-Jegher syndrome
D polycythaemia
E precocious puberty

2.177 Which of the following statements regarding adjuvant therapy of ovarian tumours are true:
A laparoscopy or laparotomy should be performed within one year of surgery for Stage I carcinoma
B chemotherapy should be used in well-differentiated Stage I carcinoma
C vincristine Actinomycin D and Cyclophosphamide (VAC) are useful in early granulosa cell tumour
D combinations of VAC, cis-Platinum and Methrotrexate have markedly improved the prognosis of malignant teratomas
E 'curative' long-term courses of alkylating agents produce leukaemia in 10% of cases

2.178 Krukenberg tumours
A occur through transcoelomic spread
B secrete oestrogens
C secrete gastrin
D contain peg cells
E are sarcomas

(*Answers overleaf*)

2.175 A **True**   20% of Stage I carcinomas of the ovary are bilateral
     B **True**   (Stage Ib) — if ascites or cancer cells are present in
     C **True**   peritoneal washings, it is Stage Ic. A mid-line incision
     D **False**   is required for adequate protocol staging. Unilateral
     E **True**   Stage I cancer may be treated by unilateral
oophorectomy in younger women as the prognosis is
much the same as for a more extensive operation but
this will greatly depend on the patient's attitude
towards fertility.

E Wiltshaw in Ref 3 Vol 1

2.176 A **True**   Thrombophlebitis migrans is associated with
     B **False**   advanced carcinoma especially ovarian malignancy.
     C **True**   Peutz-Jegher syndrome is associated with familial
     D **False**   carcinoma of the colon and ovary. Precocious
     E **True**   puberty is rarely associated with granulosa cell
tumours secreting oestrogens. Polycythaemia has
been reported associated with fibroids, but not with
ovarian tumours.

2.177 A **True**   The timing of a second-look procedure remains
     B **False**   debatable, but one year is about the right time for a
     C **False**   laparoscopy or laparotomy, otherwise false negative
     D **True**   'second looks' may be found. Chemotherapy should
     E **True**   not be used unless a recurrence is diagnozed
subsequently. VAC has been found to be useful in
late granulosa tumours and in combinations with
cis-Platinum. It has greatly improved the prognosis
for malignant teratomas. The frequency with which
alkylating agents produce leukaemia is an essential
reason why second-look procedures are performed
to exclude gross or microscopic tumour, and hence
allow these drugs to be discontinued.

E Wiltshaw in Ref 3 Vol 1

2.178 A **False**   Krukenberg tumours are secondaries (usually
     B **True**   bilateral) from primary tumours in the
     C **False**   gastro-intestinal tract. They may arise from stomach,
     D **False**   colon, gall bladder or bile duct which has
     E **False**   metastasized by lymphatic or vascular routes. They
were initially and mistakenly believed to be
sarcomata. They frequently secrete oestrogens, do
not secrete gastrin and typically have many
mucin-filled signet cells. (Peg cells are found in the
fallopian tube).

R M Feroze in Ref 4

2.179 Granulosa cell tumours
    A are Stage I in 50% of cases
    B have the features of late recurrence
    C account for 2% of solid ovarian tumours
    D produce stunting of growth
    E should be treated with surgery without chemotherapy

2.180 Ovarian cancer
    A is responsible for more deaths than carcinoma of the cervix and carcinoma of the endometrium combined (UK & USA)
    B may be detected by tumour markers
    C may be diagnozed by cytology
    D has a five-year cure rate of 80% to 90% if Stage Ia
    E most commonly arises from epithelial tissue

2.181 Hydatidiform moles
    A occur in 1:1200 pregnancies in the United Kingdom
    B characteristically secretes alpha feto protein (AFP)
    C characteristically have a trisomic chromosomal constitution
    D invade blood vessels and metastasise to the lungs
    E are associated with ovarian dermoid cysts

2.182 Choriocarcinoma
    A presents after a miscarriage
    B is treated primarily by chemotherapy
    C has a better prognosis occurring after a term pregnancy than after a molar pregnancy
    D has a prognosis related to time between antecedent pregnancy and diagnosis
    E has a 90% cure rate

2.183 Choriocarcinoma
    A is always preceded by pregnancy
    B presents with respiratory failure
    C contains chorionic villi on histological examination
    D has no intrinsic vasculature
    E must be confirmed by tissue diagnosis before commencing therapy.

(*Answers overleaf*)

2.179 A **False**   10% of solid ovarian tumours are granulosa cell
       B **True**   tumours. They are Stage I in 75–80% and should be
       C **False**   treated surgically. Chemotherapy has no place in
       D **True**   early disease but combinations such as VAC have
       E **True**   produced the occasional remission in recurrent
                      advanced cases. They are rarely malignant in
                      childhood, but produce precocious puberty and
                      hence stunting of growth.

Ref 26

2.180 A **True**   Ovarian carcinoma now accounts for 47% of deaths
       B **False**   of all gynaecological malignancies. The five-year cure
       C **True**   rate is 80% to 90% if Stage Ia, with overall Stage I
       D **True**   survival of 65–70%. The tumours cannot be detected
       E **True**   or followed by markers and 80% arise from epithelial
                      tissue.

Ref 26

2.181 A **False**   Hydatidiform mole occurs in 1:2000 or 3000 full term
       B **False**   pregnancies in the United Kingdom. Recent work on
       C **False**   the chromosomal make up shows XX pattern of sex
       D **True**   chromosomes both being of paternal origin. Triploid
       E **False**   69 composition is also seen. Benign mole
                      metastasises to the lungs and it is associated with
                      theca lutein cysts of the ovary which resolve after
                      treatment.

J S Scott in Ref 4

2.182 A **True**   Choriocarcinoma has a good prognosis (90% + cure
       B **True**   rate) using chemotherapy — usually Methotrexate
       C **False**   and/or actinomycin D. The prognosis is related to
       D **True**   age, preceding type of pregnancy, time interval
       E **True**   before diagnosis, HCG level and extent of metastasis.
                      Choriocarcinoma is preceded by abortion in 25% of
                      cases.

C Newlands in Ref 3 Vol 3

2.183 A **False**   The rare ovarian choriocarcinoma is not associated
       B **True**   with a serious pregnancy and other 'ab initio'
       C **False**   tumours occur. Although the tumour is usually
       D **True**   haemorhagic it has no intrinsic vasculature. Therapy is
       E **False**   frequently commenced without a tissue diagnosis as
                      a hormonal or radiological is adequate.

C Newlands in Ref 3 Vol 3

2.184 Oestrogen receptors
    A   are polypeptide hormones
    B   are present in all oestrogen target tissues
    C   have a reduced synthesis following oestrogen administration
    D   bind anti-oestrogens such as clomiphene
    E   can be measured to predict the response of breast and
         endometrial cancer to hormone therapy

2.185 Endometrial carcinoma
    A   is Stage II if it involves the bladder or rectum
    B   should be treated by a Wertheim's hysterectomy if it is
         Stage II
    C   occurs more commonly in urban dwellers
    D   is less common in women who have had a delayed
         menopause
    E   is decreasing in incidence

2.186 The following statements about endometrial carcinoma are correct:
    A   the incidence in the UK is approximately 40–50/100 000
    B   the incidence in the US has increased six-fold in the last ten
         years
    C   pre-operative intra-cavity radium reduces vault recurrence
    D   it occurs in 2–5% of patients with cystic hyperplasia
    E   it occurs in 40–60% of patients with atypical hyperplasia

2.187 Cancer of the endometrium is commoner in
    A   social classes 5 than 1
    B   patients with gonadal dysgenesis
    C   post menopausal patients receiving exogenous oestrogen
         and progestogen
    D   patients with an ovarian fibroma
    E   patients with osteoporosis

(*Answers overleaf*)

2.184 A **False**   All oestrogen target organs contain intracellular
     B **True**   proteins which bind oestrogens and anti-oestrogens.
     C **False**   The highest detected amounts of receptor are in the
     D **True**   endometrium and the synthesis is increased
     E **True**   following oestrogen administration and reduced
            following administration of progestogens. The level
            of oestrogen receptor in breast and endometrial
            cancer cells corelates well with the response of the
            tumour to hormonal manipulation.

M Whitehead in Ref 3 Vol 3

2.185 A **False**   Carcinoma of the endometrium is increasing in
     B **True**   incidence and is found more commonly in urban
     C **True**   dwellers for reasons which are by no means clear.
     D **True**   Tumours involving the bladder and/or rectum are
     E **False**   classified as Stage IV and extension of the tumour to
            involve the cervix necessitates pelvic
            lymphadenectomy and removal of parametrial and
            paracervical tissue in the form of a Wertheim
            hysterectomy.

Ref 27

2.186 A **False**   The incidence of endometrial carcinoma in the
     B **False**   United Kingdom is 20-30/100 000 and there has been
     C **True**   a three-fold increase in the United States mostly due
     D **False**   to the injudicious use of unopposed oestrogen
     E **True**   therapy. Malignant change occurs in less than 0.5%
            of cases of cystic hyperplasia, but in 40–60% of cases
            of atypical hyperplasia. Cystic hyperplasia is a
            common benign response to oestrogen stimulation
            and does not initially require surgical treatment.

J W Studd & M H Thom in Ref 3 Vol 1

2.187 A **False**   Carcinoma of the endometrium is due to excessive
     B **False**   oestrogen stimulation without the anti-proliferative
     C **False**   effect of cyclical progesterone, therefore it is more
     D **False**   common in the anovulatory syndrome of polycystic
     E **False**   ovary disease and less common with the inactive
            gonadal dysgenesis (unless oestrogen therapy is
            given) or an ovarian fibroma. It is more common in
            overweight, white, social class 1 patients and
            probably the other parts of the 'triad' i.e.
            hypertension and diabetes, are related mostly to the
            co-existant obesity. These fat patients tend to be the
            ones who do not develop severe osteoporosis.

J W Studd & M H Thom in Ref 3 Vol 1

2.188 Vault recurrence of endometrial carcinoma
  A   occurs in 10% of patients treated by hysterectomy alone
  B   is best prevented by taking a vaginal cuff
  C   can be prevented by pre-operative depot progestogen
  D   does not respond to cytotoxic drugs
  E   has a five-year survival of 20%

2.189 The following statements concerning endometrial carcinoma are true:
  A   the prognosis of adenocarcinoma co-existent with a hyperplastic endometrium is better than that juxtaposed with atrophic endometrium
  B   the depth of invasion of the myometrium is not included in the FIGO classification
  C   adeno-squamous carcinoma has a worse prognosis than adenocarcinoma
  D   adenocarcinoma is more common in patients with Stein Leventhal syndrome
  E   arias Stella reaction is suggestive of early endometrial malignancy

2.190 In endometrial carcinoma
  A   the ovaries are involved in 5% of cases
  B   pelvic lymph nodes are involved at the time of surgery in 10–20% of cases
  C   posterior fornix aspirate cytology is a useful screening procedure
  D   pre-operative radium reduces vault recurrence from 10% to 2%
  E   an extended hysterectomy removes the need for pre-operative radium

2.191 Uterine sarcoma
  A   accounts for 7–10% of all malignancies of the uterine corpus
  B   is commonest after the age of 50
  C   should be treated by surgery alone
  D   may be a mixed mesodermal tumour
  E   may be a hemangiopericytoma characterized by low grade malignancy.

(Answers overleaf)

2.188 A **True**   If endometrial carcinoma is treated by a
       B **False**   hysterectomy alone a vault recurrence occurs in
       C **False**   approximately 10% of patients. However this can be
       D **True**   prevented by pre-operative intra-cavity radium,
       E **False**   post-operative vault radium or the excision of a
                        vaginal cuff. Current thought is along the lines that as
                        some radiation will probably be required if the
                        myometrium is invaded, an extended hysterectomy
                        with a vaginal cuff is unnecessary. Such a recurrence
                        may respond to progestogens, irradiation or radical
                        surgery but not cytotoxic drugs. The five-year
                        survival is less than 10%

2.189 A **True**   The Arias Stella reaction in the endometrium
       B **True**   suggests early pregnancy and can be mistaken for
       C **True**   carcinoma. There is no difference in prognosis with
       D **True**   the squamous metaplasia of adeno-acanthoma but
       E **False**   the prognosis is worse with an adenosquamous
                        carcinoma and if the surrounding endometrium is
                        atrophic. Failure to consider depth of invasion is a
                        weakness in the FIGO classification.

Ref 28

2.190 A **True**   Posterior fornix cytology is not a good method of
       B **False**   diagnosis and even the value of intra-uterine cell
       C **False**   sampling is doubted. The ovaries are involved in 5%
       D **True**   and studies of Wertheim hysterectomy specimens
       E **True**   show pelvic node involvement in less than 10% of
                        cases. Vault recurrences occur in 10% of cases unless
                        an enlarged vaginal cuff is cut or pre-operative
                        intra-cavity radium or post hysterectomy vault
                        radium is applied. It is probable that the planned use
                        of radium obviates the need for an extended
                        hysterectomy.

R M Feroze in Ref 4

2.191 A **False**   Uterine sarcomata account for less than 5% of uterine
       B **True**   tumours occurring usually after the age of 50.
       C **False**   Surgery should be supported by chemotherapy
       D **True**   because of the frequency of blood-borne metastases.
       E **True**   It may be a mixed Mullerian duct (or mixed
                        mesodermal) tumour with the traditional bad
                        prognosis or the rare, but less malignant,
                        hemangiopericytoma. There are many other 'pure
                        homologous', 'pure heterologous' or mixed
                        sarcomata.

Ref 25

2.192 Recurrent endometrial carcinoma
  A   rarely affects the lungs
  B   is treated with 50 mg Medroxyprogesterone daily
  C   responds to cytotoxic therapy
  D   characteristically occurs in the lower third of the vagina
  E   is more common with adenoacanthomas than adenocarcinomas

2.193 Carcinoma of the fallopian tube
  A   usually occurs in pre-menopausal women
  B   is bilateral in 5% of cases
  C   50% are sarcomas arising from the muscularis of the tube
  D   responds to progestogen
  E   produces a positive Pap. smear

2.194 The following statements about cytotoxic drugs are appropriate:
  A   6 Mercaptopurine is an anti-metabolite
  B   Melphalan is an alkylating agent
  C   Cis-Platinum vomiting is treatable with cannabis
  D   5 Fluorouracil is a good single agent drug
  E   Methrotrexate causes stomatitis.

2.195 Cis diamine dichloroplatinum (Cis-platinum)
  A   is neurotoxic
  B   has increased nephrotoxicity when used with an amino-glycoside
  C   is cardiotoxic
  D   causes alopecia
  E   is administered intravenously

2.196 The following items are useful for the prevention of the side effects of chemotherapy:
  A   full body irradiation
  B   folinic acid
  C   scalp cooling
  D   corticosteroids
  E   leucocyte transfusion

(*Answers overleaf*)

2.192 A **False**   Recurrent carcinoma of the endometrium affects the
    B **False**   vault and the lower third of the vagina, also the pelvic
    C **False**   side wall and secondaries to lung and bone.
    D **True**   Medroxyprogesterone is useful in a higher dose of
    E **False**   100–300 mg daily. Radiotherapy is also effective for
                    pelvic masses, but cytotoxic therapy is disappointing.

R M Feroze in Ref 5

2.193 A **False**   This rarest of carcinomas of the genital tract accounts
    B **True**   for less than 0.1% of carcinomas in the pelvis. It has
    C **False**   many similarities to carcinoma of the endometrium
    D **True**   — which as an adenocarcinoma occurring in
    E **True**   postmenopausal women — may respond favourably
                    to progestogen and exfoliate cells which may be
                    detected by a Pap. smear. It may produce pain in
                    combination with a profuse watery discharge.

Ref 26

2.194 A **True**   6 Mercaptopurine is a purine anti-metabolite and
    B **True**   Methotrexate a folic acid anti-metabolite. They both
    C **True**   produce dermatitis. 5 Fluorouracil is a pyramidine
    D **False**   anti-metabolite and is a poor single agent drug.
    E **True**   Melphalan is an effective alkylating agent sometimes
                    used in combination for carcinoma of the ovary.
                    Cis-Platinum causes renal failure and also very
                    distressing vomiting which can be controlled with
                    cannabis.

B Benigno in Ref 3 Vol 2

2.195 A **True**   Cis-platinum is a heavy metal compound which
    B **True**   should be administered intravenously after prior
    C **False**   hydration in order to minimize renal toxicity.
    D **False**   Symptoms of neurotoxicity such as numbness,
    E **True**   paraesthesia and pain particularly in the fingers are
                    indications to discontinue treatment.

B Benigno in Ref 3 Vol 2

2.196 A **False**   Prophy lactic folinic acid and a scalp cooling helmet
    B **True**   effectively delay the general and local scalp side
    C **True**   effects of anti folate drugs. Irradiation and
    D **False**   corticosteroids do not help and transfusions of
    E **False**   leucocytes are used for treatment of infection
                    following a granulopaenia rather than planned
                    prophylaxis.

2.197 Convincing remissions occur with cytotoxic drugs in the following tumours:
A   carcinoma of the Fallopian tube
B   carcinoma of the vulva
C   squamous carcinoma of the vagina
D   vulval melanoma
E   ovarian secondary from a colon primary

2.198 Which of the following statements concerning chemotherapy are correct:
A   Adriamycin causes cardiac arrythmias
B   Vincristine causes peripheral neuropathy
C   Methotrexate causes haemorrhagic cystitis
D   Chlorambucil is an alkylating agent
E   Cis-Platinum produces renal failure

2.199 The following statements about pelvic exenteration are appropriate:
A   metastases outside the pelvis are an absolute contra-indication to pelvic exenteration
B   the five year survival rate following pelvic exenteration is no higher than 20%
C   pelvic exenteration is contra indicated following total dose irradiation
D   exenteration is most frequently performed for recurrent ovarian carcinoma
E   the ureters are usually transplanted into a loop of colon

2.200 Which of the following statements about malignancy in pregnancy are true:
A   cancer of the cervix in the third trimester is an indication for a classical Caesarean section
B   positive cytology should be investigated by colposcopy and cone biopsy
C   carcinoma of the cervix in the first trimester should be treated by suction curettage, followed by radiotherapy
D   the prognosis for melanoma is worse during pregnancy
E   the prognosis for breast carcinoma is unchanged during pregnancy

(Answers overleaf)

2.197 A **False**   In gynaecological oncology only choriocarcinoma
      B **False**   and ovarian tumours have hopeful remissions with
      C **False**   chemotherapy. Even ovarian secondaries from the
      D **False**   breast may undergo remission, but not from the
      E **False**   colon.

Ref 26

2.198 A **True**   It is important to know the side effects of the very
      B **True**   powerful drugs used in oncology. Cardiac
      C **False**   arrhythmias, myocardial infarctions and
      D **True**   cardiomyopathy are important and fatal side effects
      E **True**   of Adriamycin. Peripheral neuropathy is a common
                     side effect of Vincristine. Haemorrhagic cystitis is a
                     complication of the alkylating agents Chlorambucil
                     and Cyclophosphamide. The danger of renal
                     insufficiency and intractable nausea following
                     cis-Platinum may be minimized by pre-treatment
                     hydration.

C Hudson in Ref 3

2.199 A **True**   Pelvic exenteration was introduced by Brunschwig in
      B **False**   1948 and is usually performed for advanced or
      C **False**   recurrent cervical carcinoma which is confined to the
      D **False**   pelvis. With good patient selection the five year
      E **False**   survival rate is variously reported between 20–60%.
                     Although the morbidity is increased in patients who
                     have had previous irradiation, the operation is often
                     performed for persistent disease following radiation
                     therapy. The ureters are usually transplanted into a
                     loop of ileum.

R G Symonds in Ref 26

2.200 A **True**   Colposcopy and colposcopically directed punch
      B **False**   biopsies should be used for investigation of
      C **False**   abnormal cytology in pregnancy. A cone biopsy
      D **False**   should be avoided because of haemorrhage. An early
      E **True**   invasive carcinoma should be treated in the first
                     trimester by preliminary radiotherapy and if it is
                     diagnozed in the third trimester delivery of the baby
                     should be by classical Caesarean section. The
                     prognosis of breast carcinoma or melanoma is
                     unchanged by pregnancy.

Ref 26

2.201 Lymph node biopsy is indicated as a guide to subsequent therapy in the following clinical problems:
- A vulval carcinoma
- B primary surgery for ovarian carcinoma
- C endometrial carcinoma
- D second look laparotomy for ovarian carcinoma
- E pelvic exenteration.

2.202 A 'second look' operation
- A is usually performed to diagnose recurrence of cervical carcinoma
- B is usually performed in a patient without clinical evidence of disease
- C enables leukaemia to be avoided
- D should inspect the lower surface of the diaphragm
- E is preferably performed by laparoscopy

2.203 The following statements about rare ovarian tumours are appropriate:
- A Sertoli-Leydig cell tumours may have a virilizing effect
- B gynandroblastomas occur in children
- C gonadoblastomas have a good prognosis
- D Burkitts lymphoma is a common cause of ovarian swelling in Africa
- E Brenner tumours characteristically co-exist with dermoid cysts

(*Answers overleaf*)

2.201 A **True**   Para-aortic and iliac lymph node biopsies are
       B **True**   required for the management of ovarian carcinoma.
       C **False**   With primary surgery it is necessary for protocol
       D **True**   staging and evaluating the need for further
       E **True**   chemotherapy. With a second look operation it is
                      necessary to exclude disease in lymph nodes if
                      chemotherapy is to be discontinued. Pelvic
                      exenteration will not be performed if there is any
                      lymph node disease and the presence of a positive
                      Cloquet node indicates that deep inguinal and iliac
                      dissection is required. There is no indication to
                      perform a lymph node biopsy with endometrial
                      carcinoma.

Ref 27

2.202 A **False**   A 'second look' operation is an extensive laparotomy
       B **True**   performed to diagnoze and remove (or reduce)
       C **True**   recurrent ovarian tumour in an asymptomatic patient
       D **True**   without evidence of the disease. Peritoneal washings,
       E **False**   inspection of the lower side of the diaphragm and
                      multiple peritoneal biopsies are important to
                      establish that no tumour is present in which case the
                      patient may stop the chemotherapy with its 5–10%
                      chance of inducing leukaemia. The use of
                      laparoscopy is controversial but certainly inadequate
                      to exclude residual disease.

A Singer in Ref 3 Vol 1

2.203 A **True**   Sertoli-Leydig cell tumours may secrete oestrogen or
       B **False**   testosterone in 25% of cases. If Leydig cells
       C **True**   predominate, virilization occurs. Gynandroblastomas
       D **True**   have never been described in children. Burkitts
       E **False**   lymphoma is the most common cause of ovarian
                      swelling in children in Central Africa. Brenner
                      tumours co-exist with mucinous tumours

Ref 26

2.204 The following statements about colposcopic findings are appropriate:
  A   a mosaic pattern suggests a CIN lesion.
  B   a punctate pattern suggests a CIN lesion.
  C   Warty changes are characterized by irregularly folded surface epithelium.
  D   invasive carcinoma is characterized by atypical vessel formation.
  E   CIN III is clearly delineated.

2.205 On colposcopic examination
  A   active metaplasia may have the appearance of CIN I
  B   the magnification is approximately x 50
  C   the need for tissue diagnosis is obviated
  D   the transformation zone is found medial to the squamo-columnar junction
  E   the aceto-white epithelium in young patients most commonly indicated squamous metaplasia

2.206 In cervical intraepithelial neoplasms
  A   CIN I has irregular enlarged nuclei with abnormal mitoses
  B   CIN III includes severe dysplasia and carcinoma in situ
  C   CIN II does not involve the cervical glands
  D   CIN III lesions gradually blend into the adjacent normal epithelium
  E   is easily confused with active metaplasia histologically

2.207 Laser treatment for cervical CIN lesions
  A   uses carbon dioxide
  B   requires a general anaesthetic
  C   should destroy to a depth of 4 mm
  D   obviates the need for a tissue diagnosis
  E   has a higher cure rate than a cone biopsy

(*Answers overleaf*)

2.204 A **True**   Colposcopy reveals the capillary pattern on the cervix
    B **True**   and hence gives the guide to underlying pathology.
    C **True**   Both a mosaic and a punctate capillary pattern
    D **True**   suggests cervical intra-epithelial neoplasia which if
    E **True**   CIN III is usually clearly delineated from the
surrounding normal tissue. Invasive carcinoma is
characterized by an irregular friable surface as well as
atypical vessels. Warty changes are now being
recognized more frequently and may be recognized
by either a raised flat epithelium on an irregularly
folded surface, decribed as being similar to the sulci
of the brain.

J A Jordan in Ref 3

2.205 A **True**   Colposcopy with a magnification of up to 25 indicates
    B **False** the type and the extent of CIN lesions but a tissue
    C **False** diagnosis is always required before treatment. The
    D **False** transformation zone of metaplasia is lateral to the
    E **True**   squamous columnar junction and stains aceto-white.
In young patients (aged less than 20) aceto-white
epithelium usually represents squamous metaplasia
but pathology is more likely in the over-20 age group.
Similarly, aceto-white active metaplasia may easily
be mistaken for a CIN lesion.

J A Jordan in Ref 3

2.206 A **True**   CIN III contains abnormal cells and nuclei but the loss
    B **True**   of polarity is only partial. CIN II does not involve
    C **False** glands and CIN III including severe dysplasia and
    D **False** carcinoma in situ accepts that both have the same
    E **False** sinister importance. The histological division
between CIN III and normal tissue is usually abrupt
and there should be no mistaking active metaplasia
histologically although a confusion can occur both
cytologically and colposcopically.

M Coppleson & E C Pixley in Ref 27

2.207 A **True**   Laser treatment for cervical CIN lesion uses CO_2 and
    B **False** is better than cryocautery as a depth of 7 mm is
    C **False** required to ablate the lesion. The laser does not need
    D **False** any anaesthetic. A tissue diagnosis is still necessary
    E **False** before therapy, but the cure rate remains
approximately 90%, slightly lower than cone biopsy
but it can be repeated.

J A Jordan in Ref 3

2.208 Micro-invasive carcinoma of the cervix
  A   is Stage I (A)
  B   has lymph node involvement in 2-5%
  C   should have a Wertheim hysterectomy
  D   is defined by FIGO as invasion 3 mm or less below the basement membrane
  E   occurs only within the transformation zone

2.209 Stage lb carcinoma of the cervix (FIGO 1974)
  A   is carcinoma in situ with early stromal invasion
  B   has pelvic lymph node involvement in 10%–20% of cases
  C   has a five-year cure rate of 95% by surgery, radiotherapy or combination of both.
  D   has a good correlation of positive lymphograms with histologically proven lymph node metastasis
  E   has a five-year survival rate of 20% if lymph nodes are involved

2.210 The following statements concerning colposcopy are true:
  A   leucoplakia becomes visible after acetic acid application
  B   immature squamous metaplasia mimics neoplasia
  C   the squamo-columnar junction is usually visible at the external os
  D   trichomonal infection produces a punctate vascular pattern
  E   the transformation zone is absent in virgins

2.211 Terminal carcinoma of the cervix
  A   is often relatively painless
  B   usually has liver and/or lung secondaries
  C   may require urinary diversion
  D   may be helped by intrathecal phenol injections
  E   may be offered pelvic exenteration if painful

2.208 A **True**   The pathology and treatment of micro-invasive
      B **False**   carcinoma remains controversial. The FIGO staging
      C **False**   does not give clear guidance on pathology.
      D **False**   Treatment varies but the majority view would now
      E **False**   support conservative therapy as lymph node
                     involvement is less than 2%. This would usually be a
                     cone biopsy or laser vaporization. Lesions occur
                     outside the transformation zone.

R M Richart in Ref 27

2.209 A **False**   Early stromal invasion in Stage Ia (micro-invasion)
      B **True**   Stage Ib has a 15% lymph node involvement and a
      C **False**   prognosis of 80–90% regardless of modality of
      D **True**   therapy unless the nodes are involved in which case
      E **False**   prognosis is 35–55%. Positive lymphograms
                     correlate well with positive nodes but negative
                     lymphograms are not helpful.

I A Duncan in Ref 3

2.210 A **False**   With application of acetic acid squamous metaplasia
      B **True**   often mimics CIN I or II. The transformation zone is
      C **True**   the area of squamous metaplasia where the
      D **True**   columnar epithelium has been transformed into
      E **False**   squamous and is present on virtually every cervix.
                     Leukoplakia is a colposcopic and naked eye white
                     appearance before acetic acid application and
                     suggests that there might be underlying pathology.

J A Jordan in Ref 3

2.211 A **False**   Terminal carcinoma of the cervix involves the pelvic
      B **False**   nodes, parametrium and pelvic sidewall and
      C **False**   uncommonly allows the easy demise of lung, liver or
      D **True**   brain secondaries. It is therefore very painful and
      E **False**   procedures which merely prolong the distress are not
                     indicated. Exenteration and urinary diversion have a
                     place in early mid-line recurrences. The cure rate
                     following exenteration may be as high as 20% in
                     selected cases of recurrent disease — but not in
                     painful terminal disease.

Ref 26

2.212 Occult carcinoma of the cervix is:
A stage IA
B micro-invasive carcinoma
C best treated by a cone biopsy
D found incidentally in a surgical specimen following hysterectomy
E frequently associated with negative cytology

2.213 The following operative steps are taken during a radical hysterectomy:
A the lymphatic dissection is continued as far as the deep inguinal ring
B the dissected iliac nodes are reflected medially
C the common iliac nodes are removed
D the ureter is dissected free of the broad ligament from the bifurcation of the common iliac vessels to its entry into the bladder
E the uterine vein is ligated deep to the ureter

2.214 The following statements about Wertheim hysterectomy are appropriate:
A suction drainage of the pelvic floor reduces the incidence of lymphocyst formation
B bladder atony is the commonest post operative complication
C the obturator nerve is rarely seen
D the superior vesical artery is identified as a terminal branch of the internal iliac artery
E the genito-femoral nerve is frequently damaged

2.215 If Stage I carcinoma of the cervix is treated by Wertheim hysterectomy:
A the ovaries should also be removed
B the operative mortality is less than 1%
C a longitudinal incision should be used.
D para aortic nodes should be removed.
E the roof of the ureteric tunnel should always be divided.

2.216 If carcinoma of the cervix is treated with radiotherapy
A it reduces the incidence of positive nodes at subsequent lymphadenectomy
B it is more effective for adenocarcinoma than squamous carcinoma
C megavoltage therapy has a higher incidence of skin damage than autovoltage (220–300 Kv)
D point 'A' is in the same sagittal plane as the uterus 2 cm from the mid-line and 2 cm above the lateral fornix
E oestrogen therapy prevents atrophic vaginal changes

(Answers overleaf)

2.212 A **False**   Occult carcinoma of the cervix is invasive Stage IB
       B **False**   that is not apparent on clinical inspection. It may be
       C **False**   detected by cytology, colposcopy and biopsy or
       D **True**   even, regrettably, as an incidental finding following
       E **False**   hysterectomy if cytological screening is inadequate.
                          It is not to be confused with micro-invasive
                          carcinoma (Stage IA) which has a much better
                          prognosis.

I A Duncan in Ref 3 Vol 1

2.213 A **False**   Pelvic lymphatic dissection is continued from the
       B **True**   bifurcation of the iliac vessels to the circumflex iliac
       C **False**   vein. The lymphatic tissue is reflected medially and
       D **False**   removed en block. The uterine veins are superficial to
       E **False**   the ureters. The ureters should not be dissected from
                          the posterior leaf above the level of the uterine
                          vessels, as this compromises blood supply and leads
                          to fistula formation.

S Sakamoto in Ref 27

2.214 A **True**   Lymphocyst formation occurs in less then 2% of
       B **True**   cases if drainage is performed. Some degree of
       C **False**   bladder dysfunction occurs after most radical
       D **True**   hysterectomies, but it can usually be managed
       E **True**   medically. The obturator nerve is always identified
                          and stripped of lymphatic tissue. The genital branch
                          of the genito-femoral nerve runs in the fascial coat of
                          the external iliac artery and is frequently transected.

S Sakamoto in Ref 27

2.215 A **False**   A Wertheim's (or radical) hysterectomy may be
       B **True**   performed through a transverse incision which, if
       C **False**   necessary, may include cutting the rectus muscle.
       D **False**   The ovaries should be preserved in young women.
       E **True**   The lymph nodes removed are the obturator and
                          internal and external iliac groups. The para-aortic
                          nodes may be biopsied, but not removed entirely as
                          their involvement would infer systemic disease.

I A Duncan in Ref 3 Vol 1

2.216 A **True**   There is no difference in the five-year survival
       B **False**   between squamous and adenocarcinoma treated
       C **False**   with radiotherapy. Radiotherapy does reduce the
       D **True**   incidence of positive nodes and oestrogen therapy
       E **True**   should prevent the atrophic changes if used soon
                          after radiotherapy and coitus is encouraged soon
                          after therapy. Megavoltage therapy causes less skin
                          damage but more small bowel injury.

I A Duncan in Ref 3 Vol 1

References

1. Report on confidential enquiries into maternal deaths (1973–75) published 1979, HMSO
2. Office of population census and surveys (OPCS) Monitor 79/52
3. Progress in obstetrics and gynaecology, Vol 1–3 Studd John (ed) 1981–1983 Churchill Livingstone
4. Dewhurst C J (1981) Integrated obstetrics and gynaecology for postgraduates, 3rd edn. Blackwells, London
5. W B Saunders. Clinics in Obstetrics and Gynaecology — series
6. Munro Kerr's Operative obstetrics, 1977 P R Myerscough 1977 Bailliere, London
7. Chamberlain G V P Contemporary obstetrics and gynaecology, Northwood publications.
8. Pre-term labour. In: Eds Anderson A B M, Beard R W, Brudenell J M P M Dunn Proceedings of 5th study group of RCOG, 1977.
9. McGillivray I, Nylader P P S, Corney G 1975 Human multiple reproduction. W B Saunders, London
10. Barnes C 1974 Medical disorders in obstetric practice Blackwell, London
11. Gant N S, Worley R J 1980 Hypertension in pregnancy
12. Benson R C 1980 Current obstetric and gynecologic diagnosis and treatment Lange
13. Medicine Add-on Journal, 3rd series
14. McDonald R R 1978 Scientific basis of obstetrics and gynaecology 2nd edn Churchill Livingstone, Edinburgh
15. Chiswick M L 1978 Neonatal medicine
16. Quilligan E J, Kretchner N 1980 Fetal and maternal medicine, Wyley
17. Jolly H 1981 Diseases of children. 4th edn Blackwell Scientific Publications, London
18. Davies P A, Robinson R J, Scopes J W, Tizard J P M, Wigglesworth J S 1972 Medical care of newborn babies. Heinemanns, London
19. Hawkins D F, Elder M G 1979 Human fertility control, theory and practice. Butterworths, London
20. Novak E R, Woodruff, J D 1979 Novak's gynecologic and obstetric pathology. W B Saunders, London
21. Jordan J A & Singer A 1976 The cervix W B Saunders, London

22. Cohen J 1977 Abdominal and vaginal hysterectomy, 2nd edn Heinneman, London
23. Gynaecological laparoscopy. The report of the working party of the confidential enquiry into gynaecological laparoscopy. RCOG publications, 1978. (Eds) G V P Chamberlain J C Brown.
24. Lees D A & Singer A 1978 Wolf Medical Publications.
25. Jacobs H S (ed) 1980 Advances in gynaecological endocrinology. Proceedings of RCOG study group
26. Barber H R K 1980 Manual of gynecologic oncology. Lippincott.
27. Copplesen M 1981 Gynecologic oncology, Churchill Livingstone, Edinburgh
28. Disaia P J, Creasman W T 1981 Clinical gynecologic oncology, C V Mosby.
29. H Fox, Langley F A 1973 Postgraduate obstetrics & gynaecological pathology. Perganon Press, London